TRANSFORM YOUR MIND, TRANSFORM YOUR WEIGHT

How to Quit Yo-Yo Dieting
Using the Power of Your Mind

David Paul Powell

For permission requests, reports, questions, and discounts for bulk purchases, sales promotions, fund-raising, and educational needs, please contact David Powell: davidpaulpowell@rogers.com

First Edition.

Visit the author's website at: www.davidpaulpowell.com

Editor: David Powell.

Line edit, copy edit, and proofreading by Alethea Spiridon: www.freelanceeditor.ca

Book cover design by Jaycee DeLorenzo: www.sweetnspicydesigns.com

Book formatting: Nathanael More.

ISBN: 978-1-7751293-1-8

This book is not intended or implied to be a substitute for professional medical, physical or mental health advice, diagnosis or treatment. Never disregard professional medical advice, or delay in seeking it, because of something you have read in this book. Never rely on information in this book in place of seeking professional medical advice. Please see a physician and personal trainer before starting any diet or exercise program. Also, please see a physician if you are experiencing mental health concerns. The author is not licensed as a dietician, psychologist, or psychiatrist.

The information provided in this book is based on my experience, personality, and journey. Everyone's experience, personality, and journey is different. As such, results will vary. The author is not responsible or liable for any advice, course of treatment, diagnosis or any other information, services or products that you obtain contained in this book, and will not assume any liability whatsoever for the use of or inability to use any or all information contained in this book. You are encouraged to review the information carefully with your professional healthcare provider. Use this information at your own risk.

This book is dedicated to all the people who are struggling with their weight and self-esteem. I can only hope that by writing this book, I can help them see how special and strong they truly are.

ACKNOWLEDGEMENTS

Much appreciation to my family for all they have given me and for the wisdom they continue to impart on me.

Thanks to Rick Summers for being my "weight loss buddy" and for encouraging and supporting me all along the way.

Thanks to Dave Cherewaty for all his efforts and helpful suggestions on how to structure the book.

Thanks to Mike Brown for introducing me to his business contacts.

Special thanks to Alethea Spiridon at www.freelanceeditor.ca for all her great advice and excellent editing skills. You have not only assisted with editing, but have been an invaluable resource for a first time indie writer.
Thanks to all the friends and people who have listened to me and cheered me on.

I cannot end this without thanking the countless number of people who by sharing their personal stories and knowledge has added to my understanding of myself and the world I live in. It has made me a better writer and more importantly, a better person.

CONTENTS

TRANSFORM YOUR MIND, TRANSFORM YOUR WEIGHT

INTRODUCTION

CHAPTER 1:

THE PERFECT SCAM

In North America, the diet industry is a multi-billion dollar business. It has been reported that $50 billion a year is spent on different weight loss programs and products.[1]

There are as many weight loss solutions on the market as there are names for people who are overweight. There are belts, bands, gadgets, gizmos, special foods, magic pills, potions, and even tree bark from Africa, all of which claim to help you lose weight. Whether on the radio, TV, web ads, or in print, you see and hear the same message every day, that fast and easy weight loss is just a click or phone call away.

TRICKS OF THE TRADE: THE PERFECT BODY IMAGE

Everywhere you look, you see examples of the so-called perfect body. This image is the ripped, shredded muscle body for guys and the slim, toned yoga body for women. It's promoted as the ideal body to have if you want to be acceptable, worthy, and powerful. You see this image in movies, on billboard ads, and in magazines. The diet industry then tells you they have the answer to how you too can lose weight and achieve the perfect body.

Some ads are very cruel and deliberate in attacking people's areas of insecurity and shame. For example, there are diet ads that state they can help you get rid of your "cottage-cheese thighs" or that "muffin top" or those "flabby arms" and can shrink that "spare tire." These ads reinforce, and confirm, people's own distorted thinking that they are not acceptable and worthy enough as they are because they don't have this perfect body image. They must, therefore, go on a diet program to lose weight.

A pamphlet created by the National Eating Disorder Information Centre (nedic) for Eating Disorder Awareness Week said, "the development of eating problems is strongly linked to socio-cultural pressures. Thinness is falsely associated with beauty, health, happiness,

---

and self-control."[2] It also stated that "90% of women have some degree of dissatisfaction with their bodies."[3]

THE PERFECT CLIENT

Another technique the diet industry uses to convince you they can help you achieve the perfect body is to use before and after pictures. They will show pictures of people who were once overweight and beside them an image (usually digitally enhanced) of them with the perfect body they now have. The alleged "successful clients" will give their testimonials of how they struggled all their life, trying program after program to lose weight, and finally after following this particular program they lost the weight and achieved the perfect body.

The selling point in these types of ads is that if regular people lost weight using their program, so can you. It's supposed to motivate and inspire you to believe it will work for you too! All you have to do is buy and follow their program, and you will experience the same results. Although in the small print it states results may vary.

THE PERFECT CELEBRITY CLIENT

The biggest weight loss companies don't use regular people, they use the cult of celebrity to try and sell their programs and products. Celebrities who were once "overweight" and who have now lost weight appear in the media telling everyone it's the result of following the program. They never mention the fact that they can afford home gyms, personal trainers, personal cooks, and don't forget the motivation of a multi-million dollar contract. Even with all that extra motivation and extra resources, we have still seen certain celebrities (you know who they are) lose and regain weight.

PERFECT, FAST, AND EASY RESULTS

To further play on people's pain and desperation to achieve the perfect body, a lot of ads promoting weight loss promise unrealistic results, in an unrealistic amount of time. Most ads will state that in X amount of weeks, you will achieve the perfect body. You will hear person after person, tell you the amount of weight they lost and how short of a time it took them. The big wow factor is always on how much weight was lost and how fast and easy it was.

With no fear of prosecution or penalty, you will even hear ads say you can achieve the perfect body quickly and easily by eating what you want and without having to exercise. The promise of having your problems disappear quickly and your dreams appear before your eyes is very alluring to people who desperately want to lose weight and achieve the perfect body image. Most cannot resist giving it a try even though it seems too good to be true, and we all know if it seems too good to be true, it probably is. When it comes to the promise of fast and easy weight loss, nothing could be truer.

THE PERFECT LIFE

To complete the perfect picture, these ads feed the delusion that your life will be perfect when you have the perfect body. For example, there is one ad that shows the person who lost weight all dressed up and "out on the town" with friends dancing and laughing.

In another weight loss commercial, they have the successful client riding off into the sunset in a beautiful car with a beautiful person, all set to beautiful music.

The iconic image of weight loss success and living the perfect "skinny" life is to have the client running on a beach wearing a bikini.

In the pamphlet developed by NEDIC, in the 'dispelling some myths section' was the statement, "Thinness will not guarantee health, happiness, or success."[4]

THE PERFECT DEAL

To seal the deal and remove any lingering doubts that their program/product works, their promises are all backed up by risk-free, money-back guarantees. If it did not work, why would they offer a money-back guarantee? This is the question they want you to ask yourself.

These people are not fools. There has been a lot of market research done that shows most people will not follow up on returning a purchase within the required timeframe. This is what they are banking on.

THE PERFECT LIE

Given the fact that billions of dollars are being spent on these guaranteed diet solutions, why are the obesity rates on the rise? Something does not add up. If these programs truly helped people lose weight, there would be a lot more healthy people walking around, and that's just not the case. The reality is the opposite is happening.

The stats are bleak. A joint report written by the Canadian Institute for Health Information and the Public Health Agency of Canada stated that, "Between 1981 and 2009, obesity rates roughly doubled across all age groups and tripled for youth aged 12 to 17."[5] This is why there are people who believe the diet industry needs to be regulated.

In the *Canadian Medical Association Journal*, obesity doctors who are calling for weight loss companies to be regulated made the following statement: "Before we can truly address the devastating obesity epidemic, we must first stem the centuries-old flow of snake oil.[6]

As well, one of the leading researchers in self-control and the psychology of weight loss Dr. Traci Mann stated, "diets are not effective in treating obesity. We are recommending that Medicare should not fund weight loss programs as a treatment for obesity. The benefits of dieting are too small and the potential harm is too large for dieting to be recommended as a safe, effective treatment for obesity."[7]

From the above statements it would appear that so-called weight loss solutions are causing more problems than they are solving. People who are struggling to lose weight deserve to have access to true experts, true information, and true treatment methods so they can truly help themselves, instead of harming themselves. Since some children start following diet programs in primary school, it's of the utmost importance. The consequences are too serious to allow young people to buy into the destructive methodologies and messages being promoted by most diet programs. This danger is highlighted in a statement made by Dr. Brett Taylor: "As a pediatrician, I certainly see children as young as six years old who consider themselves 'fat' (or 'stupid' or 'bad'), who have, in other words, begun the process of acquiring a negative self."[8] This negative self-image will only continue to grow larger (along with their weight) if they decide to follow a fast and easy diet program to lose weight.

CHAPTER 2:

THE LOSS OF SELF

There are a couple of diet ads that try to entice you into buying their program by stating so innocently, "What do you have to lose besides the weight?" The ugly truth is there is a lot to lose when you decide to try one of these fast and easy programs to solve your perceived problem of being overweight.

No matter how hard you try, you will not lose the weight that was promised, but you will lose most of your self-worth, self-confidence, hope, and happiness over and over again. That's because most of these weight loss programs deliver the exact opposite of what is promised. Instead of losing weight, you always end up gaining weight.

You didn't know what you were getting yourself into when you attempted your first diet program. You did so because you believed it would lead down the path of success and happiness, not down the path of failure and depression.

In an article titled, "The Diet Business: Banking on Failure," the online reporter Laura Cummings asks the question, "But with research suggesting 95% of slimmers regain the weight, does the diet industry rely on our failure to make its profits?"[9]

In another article titled, "Does dieting make you fat?" it discussed William Leith who wrote a book called, *The Hungry Years: Confessions of a Food Addict* that describes his experience with yo-yo dieting.[10] He wanted to know why he always ended up weighing more than when he started and began to investigate the diet industry.

In his search for the truth, he spoke with Dr. Traci Mann, who examined 30 long-term diet studies and found that not only did most diets end up in weight gain, but the losing and gaining weight cycle has a negative impact on the body, and was linked to cardiovascular disease, stroke, diabetes, and altered immune function.[11] They concluded that it would have been better for the people not to go on a diet at all and said, "Their weight would remain pretty much the same, and their bodies would not suffer the wear and tear from losing weight and then gaining it back."[12]

THE FOUR-STAGE DIET CYCLE OF SELF-DECONSTRUCTION

After finding myself once again overweight and depressed, I too began to wonder why after losing lots of weight did I always end up gaining my weight back, plus more.

I started dieting at the age of twelve and did not stop until the age of thirty-three. That is twenty-one years of struggling to lose weight. I was up, down, and all around. I was either attempting to start a diet, on a diet, or falling off a diet.

My whole life revolved around dieting and trying to lose weight. That is of course, until I lost the weight. Then I would stop dieting and start eating unhealthy and not exercising. When I regained weight, I would start the diet cycle all over again.

What I discovered in my many years of searching for the truth was that I had been trapped in a four-stage diet cycle of self-destruction. The cycle does include a success stage (there can be no yo-yo effect without the weight loss), but will always lead back down to failure and weight gain. It's this emotional roller coaster of losing and then gaining back even more weight that creates the extreme emotional highs and lows you have been experiencing and reacting to since you started following diet programs.

Here are the stages that make up the diet cycle of self-destruction:

The 1st stage is the Relapse Stage. This is the stage where you try to stop yourself from regaining the weight you lost, but are unsuccessful and start to lose your self-worth, self-confidence, hope, and happiness.

The 2nd stage is the Rock-Bottom Stage. This is the stage where you fall into a depression over not being able to stop yourself from regaining all your weight back, plus more, and lose most of your self-worth, self-confidence, hope, and happiness.

The 3rd and longest stage is the Long Fight Stage. This is the stage where you fight for a long time to lose all the weight you gained. As you fight to re-lose the weight, you lose and gain your self-worth, self-confidence, hope, and happiness, as you gain and lose weight.

The 4th stage, and unfortunately the shortest, is the Success Stage. This is the stage where you have lost all your weight again and regain all your self-worth, self-confidence, hope, and happiness.

SUCCESS BUT ALWAYS FAILURE

This pattern of success and failure is known as yo-yo dieting in popular media, but it's so much more than just the losing and gaining of weight. It is, as stated, a cycle of self-destruction. When you are successful at losing weight, you have feelings of self-worth, self-confidence, hope, and happiness. When you inevitably regain back your lost weight, you lose most of your positive feelings about yourself and end up in a state of depression.

You go from the euphoria of losing weight and loving yourself, to the depression of regaining weight and not liking yourself. Your feelings of self-worth, self-confidence, hope, and happiness are being pulled up and down on this emotional roller coaster as you lose and gain weight using diet programs.

It's this epic fail of regaining all the weight that you worked so hard to lose that causes you to fall into a state of depression and self-destruction. You have barely tasted the sweet nectar of success only to have it ripped from you time and time again. The climb up is slow and hard, the fall fast and tragic.

ROCK BOTTOM QUESTIONS

No matter how many times you fight to lose weight using fast and easy diet programs, you will always end up with the same result: depressed and overweight. Depression, aka rock bottom, is the place you end up when you have once again regained all the weight you lost and have become bigger than ever. It's here when you have lost all your self-worth, self-confidence, hope, and happiness, that you hear yourself ask those rock bottom questions:

- Why can't I lose weight?

- Who am I?

- How can I lose weight?

- What is my purpose?

As a result of trying over and over to achieve weight loss and happiness but instead achieving weight gain and pain, you lose yourself and no longer know who you are, what you're doing, or where you're going. You don't know why you can't lose weight permanently and continue to cause yourself such pain. This is why you ask yourself those rock bottom questions. You're desperately looking for answers so you can stop the weight gain and pain.

Up until now, the answers you have come up with to your rock bottom questions have been wrong. As you will learn, it's these false answers that have been behind your failure, pain, and self-deconstruction.

CHANGE YOUR MIND, CHANGE YOUR WEIGHT

FOLLOWING FALSE GODS

Every time you hit rock bottom, your answer to pulling yourself out was to try another get-thin-quick scheme to re-lose the weight you gained. You always turned to diet gods for the answer on how to save yourself. You believed in their gospel, that if you transform your body, you will transform yourself and your life.

All you have to do is follow their diet perfectly and you will achieve the perfect body and perfect happiness in X amount of weeks. Millions of people put their trust and faith in these promises and are ultimately betrayed.

There's a commonly referenced saying about insanity coined by an unknown wise person that states, "the definition of insanity is doing the same things over and over and expecting different results." The world of dieting fits into this definition. The time has come for sanity.

Following diet programs to achieve the perfect body image has never worked and will never work. In the words of diet and exercise guru, Susan Powter, it's time to STOP THE INSANITY. Just like you stopped believing in Santa Clause and the Easter Bunny, you have to stop believing in the diet fairies. These fairies create nightmares, not fairy tales.

When you first start a diet program, you have some self-worth, some self-confidence, some hope, some happiness, some unhealthy eating habits, and are slightly overweight. After many years of dieting, you have less self-worth, less self-confidence, less hope, less happiness, have more unhealthy eating habits and are more overweight. This is the problem with the perfect, fast, and easy diet approach and why it causes so much self-destruction—it doesn't solve the root of your problems, instead it makes your original problems worse.

Rather than focusing on attacking the root of why you

believed you needed to lose weight in the first place and what eating behaviours could be contributing to you being overweight, you focused on changing the symptom, your weight. You then listened to people that said they have the answer to your problem, but instead their answer increased the intensity and severity of your problem.

What you needed was someone to help you see that your thinking about yourself was false and to show you how you could improve your eating habits. What you didn't need was someone reinforcing the idea that you're not good enough as you are and punishing you by putting you on a restrictive diet.

The perfect, fast, and easy weight loss approach does not provide the answer to what is the root cause of your problems—it only provides the answer to the symptom which it helps create, that of being overweight. This is because these types of programs are based on lies and false information. There is no such thing as a perfect, fast, and easy solution to weight loss, there is no one perfect body image, and there is no perfect "skinny" life.

When you inevitably fail to achieve or maintain these unrealistic expectations, you end up losing yourself and gaining more weight than ever. That's why this approach to weight loss doesn't solve problems it creates problems. The proof as they say, is in the pudding. How many more years/decades will you go through the four-stage diet cycle of self-destruction?

By repeatedly going on diets to pull yourself out of rock bottom, you have been missing a golden opportunity to learn the true answers to your rock bottom questions. Every time you attempt to follow a diet program perfectly and focus on having to achieve the perfect body to feel better about yourself and life, you are preventing yourself from learning the true sources of your problems, as well as the true answers to your problems. As the author of the Harry Potter series J.K. Rowling, said, "and so rock bottom became the solid foundation on which I rebuilt my life."

BRAINWASHING

Unfortunately, learning the truth will not be so easy, because when you buy into the lies of these false diet programs they become your lies. As soon as you blindly believe their claims, you unknowingly become dependent on them to define your identity and determine your purpose.

When you believe you have to lose weight and you believe

that following a diet is the answer, your self-worth, self-confidence, hope, and happiness becomes dependent on them. This is how being overweight becomes who you are, the perfect body image becomes who you have to be, and following a diet perfectly becomes what you have to do. It's also why when you fail and regain your weight plus more and end up in a state of depression, your answers to your rock bottom questions are:

- You believe there is something wrong with you and that it's your fault you failed to lose weight.

- You believe that you are unacceptable and unworthy because you are overweight and you believe you are helpless, hopeless, and cursed because you can't lose weight.

- You believe your path to weight loss success and happiness is to perfectly follow a fast and easy diet program.

- You believe your purpose is to lose weight so you can achieve the perfect body image and live the perfect, "skinny," happy life.

This is what following and failing at diets does to you—it takes away your self-worth, self-confidence, hope, and happiness. Due to repeatedly failing at an approach that doesn't work and failing to achieve a body image and perfect life that doesn't exist, you are left feeling worthless, helpless, hopeless, and depressed. These feelings are so intense, negative, and painful that you eat to escape them and lose power over controlling your own behaviour. This is how you become dependent on food to cope with your emotions and is why you end up gaining more weight than ever.

As a result of following diet programs, you became dependent on them for answers on how to eat to lose weight, you became dependent on the perfect body image to define your self-image, and you became dependent on food to cope with your emotions. The consequences of this dependency is that you never learned the truth about yourself and life, nor, how to eat healthy and cope with your own emotions and urges. In order to break your dependency and learn the truth, you're going to have to start thinking and doing for yourself. Put another way, you're going to have to learn to become independent.

FALSE THINKING

The last time I found myself overweight and depressed I had two profound a-ha moments. The first was that following diets to lose weight does not work, and the second was that it was my false thinking about the diet approach, myself, my life, eating healthy, and exercising that was the problem.

I realized that if I wanted to change my weight for the long-term, I was going to have to change my thinking. It was this epiphany that sparked my journey into the search for the truth.

In the NEDIC pamphlet, there was a quote that said, "it's not our bodies that need changing: It's our attitudes."[13]

Psychotherapist Steven Van Beek expanded on this idea that it's our thinking that we need to change. He said, "low self-esteem is caused by believing the negative things we've been told by others, and by drawing false comparisons between who we are and who we might like to be. It tends to cover up a lot of associated issues and really means 'I can't help myself live the life I want.' "[14]

Furthermore, the obesity doctors who wrote the article calling for the weight loss industry to be regulated stated, "although experts agree that obesity management requires long-term behavioural, medical or surgical intervention, the majority of commercial weight loss providers manipulate vulnerable consumers with impunity, cultivating unrealistic expectations and beliefs."[15]

Until you learn the true answers to your rock bottom questions and change the false and destructive beliefs, values, and behaviours you developed as a result of following and failing at diets, you will continue to end up overweight and depressed. Learning the true answers to your rock bottom questions is what will give you back your self-worth, self-confidence, hope, and happiness. As I'm sure you've heard, "the truth shall set you free."

HIGHER THINKING POWERS

Due to your unquestioning belief in the perfect, fast, and easy diet approach, never did you think to ask yourself what's wrong with the approach you're using to lose weight. You just automatically blamed yourself for failing, just like you automatically believed you had to lose weight to be worthy, powerful, and happy.

Not once, did you look to yourself and think that you could

solve your own weight issues. Nor did you ever think that any other part of yourself other than your outer physical appearance was valuable. This is why you remain dependent on following diet programs to lose weight—you have not been using your higher thinking powers to learn the truth for yourself.

If you want to learn the true answers to your rock bottom questions, you're going to have to start to learn to value your mind and begin to use it to question and challenge the approach you're using along with the other false beliefs, values, and behaviours you have developed. The fact that you continue to go back and use the same old approach with the same old disastrous results is proof that when it comes to how to lose weight you have not been using your rational and critical thinking powers.

Only when you learn for yourself (using the powers of your own mind) the reasons why you repeatedly fail and end up lost, overweight, and depressed, will you be able to stop repeating the same mistakes. If you have no insight or self-understanding into why you fail, you will never learn what you have to change to be successful and happy.

Most people, including myself, start following diets when they are young and don't yet have their full rational and critical thinking powers to challenge the truth of their claims. A lot of young people (and adults) believe that if it's on television, in a magazine or on the web, it must be true and good. Their claims are taken as absolute truths and no questions are asked. As a result, you end up believing you need to lose weight to be worthy, powerful, and happy and that following a perfect, fast, and easy diet program is the answer. This is where you went wrong.

The truth is, you don't "need" to lose weight to be acceptable, worthy, powerful, and happy and following a perfect, fast, and easy diet program is not the answer. As the anthropologist and author Ashley Montagu explained, "Homo sapiens is the most educable of all living things—which means that he can learn quite as many wrong things about himself as right ones, and hence confuse himself very much more efficiently than any other creature."[16] This is what happens to a lot of people when they decide to follow diets at a young age and end up developing beliefs, values, and behaviours that lead to failure, pain, and self-destruction. This is why once you have your higher thinking powers and can think and learn for yourself, you have to rationally and critically challenge your beliefs and rationally and critically re-evaluate your values and behaviours. It's the only way you can learn and become aware of what is truly true and false and what is truly good for you and bad for you.

INDEPENDENT THINKING

To think rationally and critically means you're looking for evidence, facts, and logic that proves what the true answer is. This involves you using your higher thinking powers to question, observe, listen, research, read, reason, reflect, and experiment. You have to ask yourself, "is this belief true or false?" and "is this value good or bad?" and then use your critical thinking and evaluative powers to search for the truth. This is how you build an independent, rational belief and value system that you know for yourself is true and good.

Once you form a set of core beliefs and values, you won't change your beliefs until you see for yourself that they are false (seeing is believing) and you won't change your values and behaviour until you feel the pain and destruction they cause. Just like you won't adopt new beliefs, values, and behaviours until you learn for yourself that they are true and bring you pleasure and success.

It's the knowing what is true and false and good and bad for you (because you have learned it for yourself using your own mind), that gives you the power, confidence, and motivation to change your attitude and actions for the long-term. Knowing the truth prevents you from falling victim to the multitude of false messages telling you who you are, who you have to be, and how to live to be successful and happy. This knowledge also gives you the power to resist all the temptations that you see in your environment.

When you learn the truth about the diet approach, yourself, your life, eating healthy, exercising, and how to truly lose weight, nobody, especially yourself, will be able to tell you lies or misinformation again. You only become an independent person when your behaviour is guided by a belief and value system that is based on your own rational and critical thinking. Once you become an independent thinker who knows and understands the truth, you will be able to define yourself, find your own weight loss solution, determine your own purpose, and cope with your own emotions and urges.

TRUE KNOWLEDGE IS POWER, NOT A FLAT STOMACH

When you're finished challenging your beliefs and re-evaluating your values and behaviour, you will learn that by following and failing at diets, you developed a belief and value system that was completely wrong and upside down. What you believed was true was false; what you believed was false was true; what you valued was not valuable; and what you devalued and ignored was valuable.

After using your own rational and critical thinking powers to learn the true answers to your rock bottom questions, your new, true answers will be:

- You believe that using perfect, fast, and easy diet programs to lose weight has contributed to your failure and that it was not your fault that you failed.

- You believe you are worthy, powerful, and blessed just as you are because of who you are.

- You believe your path to weight loss success and happiness is to focus on your inner mind/body and follow your new, true, good, rational belief and value system.

- You believe your purpose is to control your inner mind/body so you can control your old, false, destructive, irrational belief and value system and live the "perfect," healthy, happy life.

These new, true answers become your new, true belief and value system. It's these new beliefs and values that you have learned for yourself are true and good that will not only make you feel positive about yourself, but will also motivate you to stop using the perfect, fast, and easy diet approach and instead, follow a rational and reasonable approach. This is what will help you lose weight.

When you learn for yourself that nothing is more valuable than your mind and that you are worthy just as you are and are powerful enough to solve your own problems, answer your own questions, create your own healthy eating and exercise plan, and cope with your own emotions, you are filled with feelings of worth, power, hope, and happiness.

After learning the truth about yourself you will intimately

relate to the first verse of the song Amazing Grace by John Hopkins: "I once was lost but now I'm found." You're found when you know that everything you are and everything you need to be worthy, powerful, hopeful, successful, and happy is found within yourself/mind, not outside of yourself. This is when you learn for yourself that beauty is only skin deep and that its what's on the inside that counts. As it states in the Bible, "salvation lies within."

This universal truth can only be revealed to you by using your own higher thinking powers to discover it. You were the one that gave your Creator-given self-worth, self-confidence, hope, and happiness away, and made it dependent on being successful at diets and achieving the perfect body image. And only you can give it back to yourself. It's your irrational thinking that got you into this mess, and it's your rational thinking that will get you out of it.

Once you learn the rational truth and form your own rational belief and value system, you will break your dependency on diet programs for answers, your body image to define your self-image, and food to cope with your emotions, and instead will depend on yourself and your powerful mind. This is where true self-confidence comes from, not from how much you weigh. As Dr. Nathaniel Branden, said in his book *The Psychology Of Self-Esteem*, "Self-confidence is confidence in one's mind—in its reliability as a tool of cognition."[17]

MENTAL FOCUS

The truth is, to change your weight, you have to change your mind. Only when you transform the beliefs and values in your mind, do you transform yourself and your behaviour. You have to learn that if you want to change how you feel and behave, you have to change your thinking. This is because your beliefs and values are what cause you to feel and act the way you do. There's no more important truth you need to learn about yourself. You have to learn that feeling good is more about thinking good than looking good.

To change your false beliefs and destructive values, you have to use your mind to learn the truth. This is where your focus needs to be if you want to learn which beliefs and evaluations create the intense feelings that trigger your destructive eating behaviours, not on following someone else's plan and someone else's body image.

To control your emotional eating, you have to be in control of what's happening inside of your mind (and body). This is why your behaviour has not changed for the long-term—you have just been focused on changing your diet and your body image, instead of changing what's going on inside your mind. If you don't change your mind, you don't change anything.

All your power lies within yourself, not outside of yourself. If you want to make your body strong, you have to make your mind strong. Your focus needs to be on developing your inner self/mind, not on your outer body. You have the power to both learn the truth and to follow the truth. You are not worthless, helpless, and hopeless—far from it. This is what you have to learn.

OUTLINE OF THE BOOK

To help you learn to use the powers of your own mind, so you can learn the true answers to your rock bottom questions and change the false and destructive beliefs, values, and behaviours you developed, this book is divided into three parts.

Part one is called diet and self-deconstruction and it's where you will learn about the four-stage diet cycle of self-destruction and why you always ended up overweight and depressed using the perfect, fast, and easy diet approach. As well, you will learn why you lost and gained your self-worth, confidence, hope, and happiness as you gained and lost weight. When you're finished going through this part, you will understand how you developed the destructive beliefs, values, and eating behaviours that are behind your failure and self-destruction.

The second part is called diet and self-reconstruction and in this section you will learn the truth about who you are and how this truth heals and empowers you. As you learn the truth about the perfect, fast, and easy diet approach, yourself and your life, you will go through the four-stages of healing. After going through the healing stages, you will forgive, accept, believe, and love yourself and appreciate your life. It's your new, true, rational self-beliefs that will create the positive healing and empowering feelings that will lift you out of depression and self-destruction, and energize you to want to eat healthy and exercise.

Also, you will learn the truth about eating healthy, exercising, and how to lose weight. This knowledge will enable and motivate you to try a new approach, and create your own healthy living plan.

Part three is called lifestyle-reconstruction and here you will learn how to cope with your destructive emotional eating habits by controlling your inner body and mind. It's here, that you will learn the true value and power of your mind and the rational truth.

In this part, you will also learn for yourself that eating healthy and exercising is a reward and not a punishment and vice versa—that eating unhealthy and not exercising is not a reward but a punishment. This will motivate you to want to eat healthy and exercise and to not want to eat unhealthy and not exercise. When you've completed this part you will have the knowledge and skills needed to control your automatic, strong, destructive emotional reactions and urges, so you can follow your healthy living plan.

Throughout each part, I will show you different techniques and therapies that will help you learn the truth, and that will help you control your emotional reactions and urges, so you can follow the truth.

Additionally, you will learn some eating and exercising techniques that will help you feel good and make you want, and like, to eat healthy and exercise.

INDEPENDENT LEARNING

To get the most out of this book you can't just read it and forget about it. When you put down the book, spend some time reflecting and thinking about what you have read. By focusing your mind and mulling over in your head what you have read is how you learn the truth for yourself. Every day you have to ask yourself your rock bottom questions and use your higher thinking powers to search for the truth.

If you don't understand the meaning of a word, look it up in the dictionary. I have learned so much and gained a deeper understanding about whatever I was trying to learn by looking up words repeatedly in the dictionary. It's usually the first place I start when I want to learn about something I don't understand. This is an example of how you can start taking control of your own learning.

You also have to reflect on your own behaviour and ask yourself why you just acted the way you did. Only you can know what you were thinking and feeling. No one else.

You are also the one that has to experiment with your eating and exercising plan to figure out what works for you and what doesn't. Just like you are the one that has to evaluate your value-choices in order to learn which ones bring you pleasure and success, and which ones bring you pain and failure. Only you can know what your experience was and how you felt. No one else.

As well, you are the one that has to do the research, reading, reasoning, reflecting, and listening to discover and come to your own conclusions about who you truly are. Only you can know who you truly are. No one else.

This is about you taking control of yourself and life, and focusing your mind on the task of learning. If you don't do the rational and critical thinking with the intention of learning the truth, then nothing will change. You will just be following again and not learning and growing.

Remember, it's only when you see and feel the truth for yourself that you will change your mind and your behaviour. I don't want you to believe a word I say without verifying the truth for yourself. You have to make thinking rationally and critically a habit, and the only way you can do this is to do it every day.

Let's begin the search for the true answers to your rock bottom questions by learning the truth about the perfect, fast, and easy diet approach, and why you failed to lose weight permanently.

- TRANSFORM YOUR MIND, TRANSFORM YOUR WEIGHT

PART ONE:

DIET AND SELF-DECONSTRUCTION

(The Taking Apart of Diet and Self)

CHAPTER 4:

THE RELAPSE STAGE

I discovered the four-stage diet cycle and learned why diets don't work by analyzing my diet history and by analyzing my diet experiences. It's important that you reflect on your own history and experiences so you can know your diet story.

When you reflect on your diet history, ask yourself how long have you been dieting for. Ask yourself how many different program/ products have you tried. Ask yourself how many times have you been successful. Then ask yourself how many times have you failed and regained the weight you lost. Write the numbers down on paper if it will help you bring the truth out into the light.

BACK TO LIFE, BACK TO REALITY

The relapse stage starts when you have that first "oh-oh" moment. It's that first moment when you realize you have gained some of your lost weight back. This happens when you first notice you can barely do up your pants, or even worse, when some "friend" tells you that "you're putting on the pounds."

When you step on the scale and confirm the weight gain for yourself, you come crashing back down to reality from your heights of success. You're upset with yourself and don't understand how you could have let this happen. The last thing in the world you want to be is overweight again.

So once again you tell yourself that you have to follow a restrictive diet and lose weight. You are highly determined and confident that you will be successful. You tell yourself that you were successful at losing weight not that long ago, so no problem.

As soon as you make your first attempt to re-lose the weight you gained, that's it—you have entered the four-stage diet cycle of self-destruction.

SETTING WEIGHT LOSS GOALS

When you weigh yourself, you figure out how much weight you have to lose. The next thing you do is figure out how fast you can lose it based on what the program says. You then set an unrealistic goal of how much weight should be lost by the end of the week, as well as how much weight should be lost by tomorrow if you're going to achieve the perfect body size in X amount of weeks.

On the day you start your diet, you tell yourself that:

- I want to lose weight.

- I will strictly follow the program.

- I won't snack or eat unhealthy.

EARLY FAILURES

Chances are on your first attempt you failed. The day starts off with great promise and hope but somewhere along the way you end up giving into your desire to eat unhealthy. The next day the same pattern is repeated.

The first several failures don't have a negative impact on your self-worth, self-confidence, hope, and happiness. There is some upset and frustration, but it's nothing serious. You still believe one thousand percent that you will be successful.

The early failures are attributed to "just a case of getting warmed-up." The next day, you hop back on the scale and count how many more pounds you gained and readjust how much weight you now need to lose every day if you want to lose X amount of weight in the time that was promised.

VALUE-CONFLICT

Unfortunately, you were unaware that you were failing due to a value-conflict that was set up within yourself as a result of following a restrictive diet program. The value-conflict is the battle between wanting to follow the program in order to lose weight but also wanting to eat the food you love. No matter what choice you make, a value will be denied. If you choose to eat unhealthy you will achieve instant gratification, but will sacrifice your value of wanting to lose weight and achieve the perfect body. If you choose to stick to the program, you will be denying yourself instant gratification, but will feel better the next day when you step on the scale. Since you are used to eating what you like (that's what caused you to regain the weight in the first place), the desire for instant gratification is strong and hard to deny.

THE MORE YOU CAN'T HAVE SOMETHING, THE MORE YOU WANT IT

As soon as you try to follow the diet program you're on, your urge to eat what you want is triggered. Whenever you're told you cannot have something, especially something you like, the more you want it. For example, this is why parenting experts tell parents not to tell their teen to stop dating someone they don't approve of. It's well-documented their teen will only end up rebelling and liking that person even more.

It's no different for food. Since you have to follow a restrictive eating program to lose weight and cannot eat the foods you love or the amount you want, it creates cravings. It makes you think about all the food you want to be eating. All day you are seeing and smelling the food you desire but can't have. Now you want the food you like more than you ever have in your entire life. By going on a low calorie/restrictive diet, it makes you want and value eating unhealthy food that much more. This is what increases the intensity of your cravings and makes it more likely that you will rebel and "go off your diet."

On a show called *Vox Talk*, they had a discussion called "The Skinny on Fat," where Nutritionist Sara Vogelzang stated, "When you're on a fad diet you become excessively concerned about the food you're eating. So, it's like if you're deprived of sleep, when you don't get enough sleep all you think about is sleep and trying to get more sleep."

UNDER PRESSURE

When you first experience cravings in the relapse stage, you give into them right away. Your cravings are strong and since you're not in the habit of fighting them, you satisfy them. As you continue to fail and regain weight, you start to put up more of a fight to stick to what the diet says to eat. You now naturally put some pressure on yourself to succeed. This is when the value-conflict really starts to intensify.

When you start to fight with yourself to follow the program and tell yourself that you can't give into your cravings, the pressure builds within. The pressure grows as you fight with yourself to stick to your diet program and not satisfy your growing cravings. It's like those old cartoons where there is an angel on one shoulder telling you to do the good and right thing and the devil on the other telling you to do the wrong and bad thing. You drive yourself crazy as you go back and forth between the two polar opposite value-choices. To eat or not to eat becomes the question.

You clench your teeth and squeeze your fists in an attempt to stick to your diet program. You keep on telling yourself you don't want to be overweight again and that you want to lose weight. With each passing second, the pressure builds within until it reaches the point where you cannot take it anymore and crumble. You end up giving in and satisfying your cravings so you can escape the pressure and resolve your value-conflict.

DEADLINE

What further adds to the pressure you feel is that you have to lose X amount of weight in X amount of weeks. All your mental focus is on that future magical date when you're supposed to reach your weight loss goal. Each passing day is marked off on the calendar until it's the final countdown.

Every day you don't lose weight, the more pressure you put on yourself to lose even more weight faster, and as a result the more intense your value-conflict becomes. You know every time you go off your diet the more likely it is that you won't lose X amount of weight in X amount of time and so the pressure increases. If you were or are in school, you know how the pressure builds when you haven't started an assignment that is almost due.

BINGE EATING

Although you put up a good fight, more times than not you satisfy your cravings so you can experience relief. After such an intense fight, when you do satisfy your cravings it's like a "shark-eating frenzy." You end up eating as much food as you can, as fast as you can. It takes a lot of food to not only satisfy your denied cravings, but also to depressurize.

Once you're stuffed and sedated, you're temporarily free from the intense, emotional conflict within. This is how people who follow diet programs become binge eaters. It's also where people learn that food is not only good for satisfying pleasure, but is also good for escaping pain. In an article titled, "Eating to numb the pain," it stated, "Many binge eaters may also have a history of going on diets and failing."[18]

IDENTITY CONFLICT

As the deadline date creeps closer and as you continue to fail and gain weight, you now tell yourself that:

- I have to lose weight.
- I have to follow the diet program.
- I can't eat unhealthy.

At this juncture, you no longer want to follow your program and lose weight; you have to. It's here that following your diet program and losing weight became value-priorities. This is how your self-worth became dependent on your body image, and how your self-confidence became dependent on following your diet perfectly. When this happened, your body image became who you are, and following a diet program and losing weight became your purpose.

You now needed to follow the diet program perfectly and lose weight to feel good about who you are. Meaning that when you don't, you lose some of your self-worth, self-confidence, hope, and happiness. This is how you lost control over defining yourself and determining how you feel and behave.

Instead of helping yourself, you are now working against yourself. You only like the ideal skinny you and not the real bigger you. You only love and reward yourself when you are following your diet and losing weight. When you don't follow your diet and lose weight, you hate and punish yourself. This causes the negative and painful emotions, which make you want to binge to escape.

You have to want to lose weight because you love the real you right now, not some ideal you in the future. The humanistic psychologist Carl Rogers said, "the greater the discrepancy between the real self and the ideal self, the more maladjusted children will be."[19] He believed it was crucial that children develop a positive self-concept.[20]

The diet approach creates a big discrepancy between the real bigger you and the ideal skinny you. This is the identity-conflict that is created and is how you put your self-worth, self-confidence, hope, and happiness in a position to be won or lost.

THE MORE YOU WANT SOMETHING, THE MORE YOU CAN'T HAVE IT

Having to be perfect just adds to the pressure you feel and makes it harder to be successful. By making losing weight a value-priority you have to achieve to feel good about yourself, you end up in the very stressful position of having to be perfect at following the program you're on. Every day and every minute becomes an epic battle that you have to win or else you lose. It's very black and white. There is no room for error—you have to be perfect. Your very selfhood and happiness is riding on it.

Whenever you have to be perfect, it creates intense stress within. You end up obsessing over the fact that you have to win. All your focus is on the results and how you have to lose weight to be worthy and happy and can't mess up.

When you have to follow a diet program perfectly, this means if you have a morsel more you fail. The stress that this high-stakes game creates becomes so intense that you feel you have no choice but to binge on food to escape.

Speaking to the harm caused by having to be perfect, writer Chuck Gallozzi wrote this in one of his wise columns: "it is not only our motivation, but our approach that can block our progress. Perfectionists, for example, set unrealistic goals. By setting them too high, they condemn themselves to failure and pain."[21]

THE BEAT DOWN BEGINS

Once you have to be perfect and lose weight, you take your next attempt very seriously. You now feel a sense of urgency and put intense pressure on yourself to succeed. All day you remind yourself that you have to stick to the diet program and lose weight.

When you unfortunately fail, how you react to this failure is different from the others. This time, you are very hard on yourself. When you step on the scale and see that you have gained back even more weight, you go ballistic.

Your earlier failures were just shrugged off. Now you yell and scream and call yourself all sorts of negative and nasty names. It's a character assassination of the worst kind. When you're done beating yourself up, you feel terrible.

TOXIC REACTION TO FAILURE

From this point on, beating yourself up and calling yourself negative and demeaning names becomes your automatic reaction to failing. Your personal attacks on yourself regarding your weight and your inability to do something about it causes you to feel the toxic emotions known by the acronym G A A S S:

G is for Guilt.

A is for Anger.

A is for Anxiety.

S is for Shame.

S is for Sadness.

Every time I didn't follow my diet program, I would experience each one of these negative, painful emotions. I would feel guilty because I broke my vow and didn't act according to the law of the diet. I would berate and verbally lash myself over and over again as if I had committed the worst sin known to humankind.

The fact that I failed and gained weight enraged me. I was angry and I would let myself have it. I would never yell at another person like I yelled at myself.

Once the anger subsided, I would then feel the anxiety of not being able to stop myself from gaining weight and ruining my life. This caused me great worry and concern.

Since I weighed even more, I felt ashamed. I felt more shame when I thought about what other people must think about me.

In the end, I was always left with a feeling of deep sadness for gaining weight instead of losing it. Afterwards, because I felt so bad about myself and my life, I would turn around and binge on more food to escape.

The toxic G. A. A. S. S. emotions increase in intensity and duration with each failure you have and with every pound you gain. You beat yourself up a little harder, yell at yourself a little louder and do it for a little longer with each failure. In order to escape the intense toxic feelings, you binge on food to escape. After every failure and beat down, you lose a little more of your self-worth, self-confidence, hope, and happiness.

Certified hypnotherapist Cathrine Moller had this to say about eating and feeling guilty: "If you want to do what you think you shouldn't want to do, then at least have peace with it. If you say, 'I shouldn't eat this chocolate,' then do so and beat myself up for having done it, it's very likely that I'm going to eat even more in order to soothe myself."[22]

Kaleb Montgomery, a practitioner of traditional Chinese medicine, made this profound statement: "My own take is that guilt (about indulgences) is worse for us than the chocolate, alcohol, or whatever."[23]

FAILURE AFTER SUCCESS

Since you continue to make daily attempts and try your best, the odds fall on your side that you will have a few successes here and there. When you have some success, you think, "This is it, I'm back in business." Unfortunately, the successes don't last long in this stage. You will sooner rather than later give into your desire to eat unhealthy and will break your winning streak and start another losing streak.

Failure after success is always more devastating. All your renewed self-worth, self-confidence, hope, and happiness quickly disappears. You are once again left upset and confused. You thought you were on your way to victory—you don't know what happened? You can't believe you blew it and failed again. Your mind is blown. You are now even more upset and beat yourself up even harder. As a result, your toxic emotions are more intense, which leads to more binge eating to escape.

TOXIC REACTION TO FOOD HANGOVER PAIN

What makes it even harder to stop yourself from regaining all your lost weight is the pain you feel when you're done binging on large amounts of food. The food hangover you feel after you're done binging is similar to the hangover people feel when they have had too much to drink. You have:

- a headache;

- a stomachache;

- a dry mouth;

- diarrhea;

- no energy;

- no mental focus.

All you feel like doing is binging on even more food to escape the pain you feel. When you feel tired or are in pain, your body craves starchy and fatty foods. These types of foods quickly replenish you and bring you temporary relief.

The way you react to this food hangover pain not only makes you gain more weight, it leads to more failure and pain, which further increases your urge to binge on food to escape.

STRESSED TO THE MAX

As you continue to fail and feel toxic G.A.A.S.S, and food hangover pain, and binge to escape, you reach the point where you feel you can no longer cope. You feel you can no longer withstand the pain and have to eat to escape. Every day you fail, the pain and your urge to binge increases.

When you know that your actions are causing you extreme pain and are ruining your life and you don't know what to do or feel like you can't do anything to stop it, it creates extreme stress. You end up becoming so overwhelmed by your situation that it triggers your fight-or-flight response. Whenever you feel your survival is in jeopardy, your fight or flight response is triggered.

This intense response is felt in your mind and body. Your mind races as it frantically searches for answers, your heart pounds, your breath quickens, and your blood pressure rises. You feel like you're going to lose control and implode. When you reach this state, you have to make a choice either to fight or take flight. Whatever choice is made, all that matters is that the threat to your survival is removed.

Since you have little self-worth or self-confidence left and are in the habit of escaping to feel relief, you take the flight option and choose to binge on food to escape. You feel it's the only choice you have if you want to survive and make it through the day. As Pamela M. Peekem MD, MPH wrote in a magazine piece about stress, "When you feel helpless and defeated, your stress hormone levels skyrocket and stay there. As a result, you can neglect or even abuse your mind and body. That's unsafe stress."[24]

As you count down toward the deadline date, you continue to fight with what little willpower you have left. Some of your attempts end early and some go right down to the wire, but all have the same result: failure, weight gain, and loss of self-worth, self-confidence, hope, and happiness.

More and more, you lose your motivation and will to fight. Most of your time is spent thinking about how bad you feel and how you should stick to your program while you do the exact opposite.

BACK WHERE YOU STARTED

As you get bigger and the date to achieve your weight loss goal gets closer, you're forced to face the painful truth that instead of losing weight, you're going to regain all the weight you originally lost. You are crushed. Your worst nightmare is coming true. You are overweight again and are back to wearing your "fat clothes."

Once your expectation of successful weight loss is shattered, so are you. You have little feelings of self-worth, self-confidence, hope, or happiness left. Instead, you feel mostly worthless, helpless, hopeless, and unhappiness. You sink further and further down until you have regained all the weight you originally lost. This is when you enter the second stage of the cycle.

CHAPTER 5

THE ROCK BOTTOM STAGE

WHY YOU GAIN MORE WEIGHT THAN EVER

In the rock bottom stage there are no more attempts. You see no point. You have worked hard for months trying to lose weight and have achieved the exact opposite results you wanted. As a result, you no longer believe you can or will ever lose weight. When you think about trying another diet attempt, you tell yourself:

- What's the point, I will only fail.

- I can't lose weight.

- I won't lose weight.

- I will never lose weight.

A psychologist named Victor Vroom created a theory called the Expectancy Theory.[25] This theory is often used by employers to try and motivate their employees to work harder. The theory states that for people to remain motivated, there has to be the expectation that their effort will lead to success and that their success will lead to the rewards they want. If there isn't this effort-success-reward relationship, the effort stops. As the theory states, they lose their motivation because they believe they will not receive the rewards they want and expect.

This is why when you don't achieve the expected results of the diet program, you quit trying. You no longer believe and trust that your effort will lead to weight loss and happiness. As a result, you're no longer motivated to put forth the effort to try and follow a weight loss program. All self-belief and hope has been lost.

LOSS OF SELF-DETERMINATION AND SELF-CONTROL

When it comes to losing weight and being overweight, you believe your fate has been sealed. You believe other forces more powerful than you have predetermined your destiny. You believe you have been cursed to this fate by the powers that be. This is what is known in psychology as having an external locus of control.

People are said to have an external locus of control when they believe that forces outside of themselves are responsible for what happens to them, regardless of what actions they might take. Conversely, people with an internal locus of control believe they are responsible for their own successes and failures. In a research paper about locus of control the authors stated that, "data indicate that health-specific internal scorers are more likely to engage in presumed health-enhancing behaviours like quitting smoking, controlling diet, doing aerobics, or engaging in 'serenity' exercises than their external counterparts."[26] This is an example of how important it is to believe you are the master of your own destiny.

By failing at diets, you lose your self-efficacy. You end up losing belief in yourself and your abilities to affect change and be successful. I heard a mixed martial arts fighter say in an interview, "there is no bigger blow to your ego than to try your best at something and still fail." Every failed diet attempt was a daily blow to your ego. Until, there was no ego left.

DEPRESSION

As a result of gaining back all the weight you lost in spite of trying your hardest, you end up developing negative, false, destructive, core beliefs about yourself and your life. You believe and tell yourself that:

- you are unacceptable and unworthy;

- you are a born failure;

- your life sucks;

- you have been cursed by a higher power to be overweight forever.

These negative beliefs play over and over in your head. All

you can think about is the weight you regained and how you will never re-lose it. You don't like yourself or like how it has negatively impacted your life. When you think about the future, all you see is doom and gloom.

You even stop wanting to go out because you don't feel good about yourself. You have zero or little self-worth, self-confidence, hope, or happiness and as result, feel worthless, helpless, hopeless, and depressed. Due to months of unhealthy eating, you also feel intense physical pain.

There was an article in *Psychology Today* that looked at the link between depression and being obese that referenced a study by Jeffery Schwimmer, M.D. of the University of California, San Diego. He says, "obese children reported scores [on a quality of life survey] were as bad as cancer patients in each and every domain of life."[27] This is a clear illustration of how crucial it is for children to have a positive self-image. It's also an indictment on society and the value that's placed on being slim.

When you feel worthless, helpless, hopeless, and depressed, it's really hard to pick yourself up off the floor and try again. This is why this time you don't and stay down for the count. These extreme, negative and destructive feelings caused by your false rock bottom beliefs combined with the feelings of extreme pain caused by your months of binge eating drive you to eat even more to escape.

Day after day, week after week, all you do is binge on food to escape. After doing this for a few weeks, it does not take long before you find yourself weighing more than ever. This is why you end up weighing more than when you first started dieting.

There does appear to be a link between being obese and being depressed. In a report by the US National Center For Health Statistics, it stated that 43% of depressed adults are also obese.[28] Given how underreported depression is, you can bet the number is even higher.

CRISIS POINT

Reoccurring thoughts of serious loss are what bring you to the last phase of the rock bottom stage: the crisis point. As you continue to overeat, you reach the point where you know you are close to crossing the line. You know that if you don't do something to stop yourself from gaining weight you're going to reach the point of no return.

When feelings of depression are so strong and the pain so

intense, it can affect your ability to function normally. It can reach the point where you don't even feel like cleaning yourself or cleaning your place. If you can, you call in sick at work or you skip classes. It becomes hard to face yourself and the world. All you feel like doing is overeating to escape how you feel. Thoughts of being fired from your job or having to drop out of school or worse, add to your intense, negative emotional state.

SUICIDAL IDEATION

The pain and unhappiness becomes so unbearable that you start to question whether your life is worth living. Since you believe there is nothing you can do to lose weight, you have thoughts of putting yourself out of your misery rather than face another day being overweight and in pain.

When you're in a state of depression and chronic pain thoughts of suicide can be normal. Both feelings of depression and feelings of worthlessness and hopelessness have been linked to suicide.[29] In one study, it was found that young teens who were obese were more likely to report having suicidal thoughts.[30] The good news is that being obese did not increase suicide attempts—those statistics were the same as the general population.[31] When suicidal thoughts become predominant, or a suicide plan starts to be formulated, it's recommended by mental health professionals that the person seek immediate medical help.

If you have, or are experiencing, suicidal thoughts and feelings you're not alone. Here's the story of actor Wentworth Miller, from the TV show *Prison Break*. He was being ridiculed on Facebook for the weight he had gained (surprise, surprise) and he bravely told his fans that he used food to help cope with depression and suicidal feelings.[32] He went on to say, "I was looking everywhere for relief/comfort/distraction. And I turned to food. It could have been anything. Drugs, Alcohol, Sex."[33]

CORE QUESTIONS ABOUT IDENTITY AND LIFE

When you start to question your existence and whether your life is worth living, that is when you start to ask yourself those rock bottom questions:

- Why can't I lose weight?
- Who am I?
- How can I lose weight?
- What is my purpose?

It's here that a decision must be made: Are you going to sink into the abyss and lose everything, or are you going to rise out of the ashes? Being the true fighter that you are, you choose to start the battle of the bulge all over again.

THE CYCLE CONTINUES

Once again, your answer to climbing out of rock bottom is to go on a perfect, fast, and easy diet program to lose weight. Driven by pain and desperation, you gather up what little energy and willpower you can, close your eyes, plug your nose, and jump back on the diet merry-go-round. This is when you enter the third stage.

THE LONG FIGHT STAGE

WHY IT TAKES SO LONG TO RELOSE THE WEIGHT

Since you're starting from rock bottom, losing weight is now harder than ever. Not only do you weigh more than ever, you're in a state of depression and pain and have little self-worth, confidence, hope, or motivation to fight with.

To add to the difficulty is the fact, that since you have been binging on food to escape your negative emotions and pain for so long, it has become a strong habit. There seems to be a consensus amongst most "experts" that it takes around three weeks to establish a habit. The longer you do the behaviour, the stronger the habit and the harder it is to break.

It's a common reaction to soothe negative feelings and pain not only with drugs and alcohol but with food as well. For example, this is why in the movies or on TV, you often see the person eating ice cream after a break up. As explained by Dr. Valarie Taylor in an article about stress and food cravings, "when people are depressed, when they're stressed, their serotonin levels are decreased. So when you talk about comfort food, it actually is that—it's comforting. When people eat it, you get a burst of serotonin. That makes you feel happier."[34]

I know by the time I hit rock bottom I felt I had no choice but to overeat. The feelings of depression and pain were so intense that I didn't think I could make it through the next second, let alone the whole day without binging to escape. As stated in Bellwood's Eating Disorders Recovery Program pamphlet: "Some people develop eating disorders to cope with stressful and emotional situations that are too painful or difficult to address directly."[35] This is how eating/binging becomes the way you cope with negative feelings and pain.

DESTRUCTIVE EMOTIONAL EATING HABITS

As you have learned by going through the relapse and rock bottom stage, the perfect, fast, and easy diet approach by its very design of food/calorie restriction, unrealistic expectations, and perfect body worship creates an extreme, intense, toxic emotional environment of inner conflict, cravings, pressure, and stress that makes it harder for you to lose weight and easier for you to gain weight. When you inevitably fail and gain weight, you start to feel toxic guilt, anger, anxiety, shame, sadness, and eventually worthlessness, helplessness, hopelessness, and depression. In order to cope with these extreme, intense, destructive feelings, you develop a lot of destructive emotional eating behaviours.

To make matters worse, the pain caused by overeating to escape makes you want to eat even more. This is what happens to you when you follow perfect, fast, and easy weight loss programs. It actually makes you develop destructive emotional eating habits to escape the destructive, intense, extreme emotions and pain it creates.

Talk about sleeping with the enemy. What a set up for failure and self-destruction. The very action you have to do to achieve the perfect body in order to feel good about yourself (not overeat), you become dependent on to relieve yourself from all the cravings, negative emotions, and pain created by following and failing at the perfect, fast, and easy diet approach. As a result, you become a:

- PLEASURE EATER - Whenever you can't have the food you love, your cravings are triggered. You end up liking and wanting the food you love more than ever.

- ALL-OR-NOTHING EATER - As soon as you fall off a diet, you're triggered to eat as much of the food you love until you start your next attempt.

- PRESSURE EATER - When you want to stick to your diet and lose weight but also want to satisfy your cravings, you're triggered to binge to escape the pressure caused by your value-conflict.

- TOXIC G. A. A. S. S. EATER - When you fail and beat yourself up and feel bad about yourself, you're triggered to eat to escape.

- FOOD HANGOVER/PAIN EATER - When you feel the pain of overeating, you're triggered to eat to escape.

- WIN-OR-LOSE EATER - When you don't follow the diet program perfectly, you are triggered to eat unhealthy for the rest of the day.

- STRESS EATER - When you have to eat perfect to feel good about yourself but feel like you can't, you're triggered to binge to escape.

- DEPRRESSION EATER - When you regain all your weight back and feel bad about yourself and life, you're triggered to quit and binge to escape.

- BINGE EATER - You're triggered to eat a lot of food, both to satisfy intense cravings and to escape intense negative emotions and pain.

- NIGHT TIME EATER - When you fight your intense feelings and cravings all day, you're triggered to eat so you can calm yourself down and go to sleep.

- NO BREAKFAST EATER - When you binge late in the evening, you don't feel like eating in the morning.

It's due to all of these dysfunctional and destructive emotional eating habits you develop that it takes so long for you to re-lose the weight again. Now to lose weight and make it back to the success stage, you have to fight through each one of these destructive eating habits. As soon as you break one bad eating habit, you're confronted by another. When it comes to following diet programs to lose weight, the only thing that is fast and easy is the gaining of weight, not the losing of it.

STEPS FORWARD AND STEPS BACKWARD

You become so used to escaping negative and painful feelings by binging on food, that when you try to follow a diet program, you can't. You don't feel you can make it through a day without binging on food to escape the depression, distress, and despair you feel. You tell yourself that you can't take the stress of having to eat perfect but wanting to do the exact opposite which is to binge on food to escape.

When you first start to follow a diet program in the relapse stage, you fail because you are not used to denying yourself immediate gratification. When you first start a program in the long fight stage, you fail because you are not used to denying yourself immediate relief from pain.

The value-conflict you face in the long fight stage is more intense because not only are the two values complete polar opposites, they both demand an immediate response. You urgently have to follow your program perfectly to stop the pain, but you also urgently have to binge on food to escape the pain. Since you're already in distress, it doesn't take much to trigger your flight response.

As a result, in the beginning, sustained success is a rare occurrence and you're still gaining more weight than you're losing. You have the odd winning streak here and there, but that is followed by an even longer losing streak. After each failure, you're knocked back down into rock bottom mode and it takes awhile before you even think about making another attempt.

You can repeat this pattern of failing for a long time. Every time you take a step forward, you take two or three steps backward.

BATTLING

As you fight on trying to cope with all your destructive emotional eating habits and stick to your diet, you experience a long emotional roller-coaster ride of losing and gaining your self-worth, self-confidence, hope, and happiness as you gain and lose weight. When you have some success, you feel good about yourself and think you're on the road to success. When you fail, you feel bad about yourself and hit rock bottom.

As you courageously continue to pick yourself back up off the floor, you become stronger and your winning streaks become longer. You bravely and miraculously fight your way out of depression and stress through sheer willpower alone.

When you fail you might still beat yourself up, feel toxic G.A.A.S.S., and go down for awhile, but you no longer quit and hit rock bottom. The winning streaks and weight loss have proven to yourself that you can be successful. The self-belief and positivity that you have gained is enough to propel you forward.

BREAKTHROUGH

Now your successful attempts start to outnumber your failures. The winning increases your self-worth, self-confidence, hope, and happiness. This gives you more power and motivation to fight and break all your destructive emotional eating habits. Since most of your bad eating habits were developed to escape negative and painful emotions, when you feel more positive and powerful there is less of an urge or need to escape.

Less and less time is spent on thinking about having to follow your program and more and more time is spent on just doing it. You're now in the habit of following your program on the regular and have the momentum of "winning" on your side.

After a failure, you bounce back quick, usually the next day. When you step on the scale and see that you have gained weight, you are determined to re-lose it. There's no more beating yourself up and feeling toxic G.A.A.S.S.

Once you have lost a significant amount of weight and are thinking and feeling more and more positive about yourself and life, you know you're on your way to reclaiming your dream.

IN THE ZONE

When you enter the zone, all you have is success. There are no more failures. You are in the daily habit of following your diet and no longer have to fight with yourself to do it. You no longer even have to think about it—it has become automatic.

The pounds continue to drop off, and eventually you lose the weight you regained. When you're wearing your "skinny"jeans, you know you have achieved success.

CHAPTER 7:

THE SUCCESS STAGE

SWEET VICTORY

The success stage is the stage where you raise your arms in victory. You have won the long fight and have achieved your dream of an acceptable, worthy, and powerful body/self-image. All you have left to do is some touch-up work and lose "the last ten pounds."

You look great and you feel great. Now that you're weighing the right weight and wearing the right size, you love and have confidence in yourself again. You feel like you have just climbed Mount Everest and are "king of the world." You feel like you can do anything and that anything is possible. Your internal locus of control has been restored.

You wake up and bounce out of bed full of energy, enthusiasm, and excitement at the anticipation of having a great day. Instead of being in a state of depression as you were in rock bottom, you're in a state of euphoria.

CHANGING YOUR VALUE PRIORITIES

Now that you're no longer overweight and in pain, achieving the perfect body image and following a diet is no longer a priority. You no longer weigh yourself or focus on how much weight you have to lose. All your focus is now on experiencing pleasure and living the perfect, "skinny," happy life.

Every time I would lose a lot of weight, the first thing I would do is go out and buy new clothes. I would then call some friends to go out with. I wanted to be seen out on the scene looking good. Every chance to go out and attend a social event, I was there. This meant that most weekends I was out with people and sometimes during the week as well.

My focus was now on my positive body image and positive

life, rather than my negative body image and negative life. I was now being driven by pleasure instead of pain.

RESTING ON YOUR LAURELS

In the beginning, when you first host or attend social functions, you decline to have any unhealthy food or drinks. While everyone else indulged, you refrained. This is because you were still in the habit of following your diet.

After a month or two in the success stage, when you are again offered unhealthy food and drinks, you think to yourself, "Why not?" and tell yourself:

- I deserve to treat myself.

- A little bit won't hurt.

- Everybody else is having some.

- I have everything under control.

- I will never regain my lost weight.

You end up talking yourself into partaking and after you have a great time with everyone eating and drinking, you now want to do it again. It's for this reason, that it's not long before you convince yourself that the odd day here and there (whether in a social setting or at home) eating and drinking unhealthy is okay. As Microsoft founder Bill Gates said, "success is a lousy teacher, it seduces smart people into thinking they can't lose."

CAUGHT UP

Although you're not aware of it, this is the beginning of the end. Soon the odd day of eating unhealthy turns into a few times a week. Every time you go out with friends, attend a family function, or are tempted at home, you indulge in unhealthy food and drinks. Before you know it, following your diet is no longer a part of your daily routine.

You're still fitting into the same clothes and are still feeling good, so you think everything is great. In your head you're still living the dream. In reality, you're gaining weight and have lost your momentum and habit of following your diet.

After awhile, you're unhealthy lifestyle choices start to catch up with you. You start feeling food hangover symptoms and no longer feel like sticking to your diet. Unbeknownst to you, you're back in the habit of eating unhealthy.

Not until you become aware that you have gained weight will you again be motivated to follow another diet program. Once you do, you re-enter the relapse stage and start the cycle all over again.

WHY YOU START TO REGAIN WEIGHT

The reason you always start to regain your lost weight in the success stage is because you have not changed your belief and value system. You have not learned the truth about yourself nor the value of eating healthy. When you were following a diet, you were not doing it because it was good for the real you. You were only doing it because you were told that's what you had to do if you wanted to achieve the ideal you. As a result, eating healthy became a means to an end. You ended up seeing eating healthy as the price you have to pay to have the perfect body and be happy. It was a necessary evil. You saw it as a form of pain and punishment and not the pleasure and reward that it really is.

This is why once you achieve weight loss success, you quit dieting and go back to eating unhealthy. Since you lost weight and gained back your self-worth, self-confidence, hope, and happiness, you lost your motivation to follow the diet program you were on. There was no longer any reason to—you achieved what you wanted. As a result, you let down your guard and eventually went back to doing what you like, which is to eat unhealthy and not exercise. Nobody is going to continue to do what they don't like to do, if they don't have to.

Due to following restrictive, unrealistic, unhealthy diet programs, you never learned the value of eating healthy or how to do it. You were either following a restrictive diet program or you were binging. There was no moderation or middle way. It was either extreme depravation or extreme excess. You have to learn to eat in a way that is rational and realistic. When you learn how to truly eat healthy, instead of feeling starved or stuffed, you will feel pleasure and power.

CHANGING YOUR BELIEFS
AND VALUES

If you want to stay in the success stage, you're going to have to change your beliefs and values. In order for this to happen, you have to learn for yourself that eating healthy is pleasurable and that eating unhealthy is painful. When you learn this, you will adopt eating healthy as a valued lifestyle you want to live, not one that you have to live to lose weight.

Before you can learn to believe in and value eating healthy as a way of life, you have to learn to believe in and value yourself/mind. You have to change your reason for wanting to lose weight and learn to accept and love yourself as well as your life just as it is today. You have to learn that you're acceptable, worthy, powerful, and blessed without the weight loss. This is where true feelings of worth, power, hope and happiness/pleasure come from. Once you learn the truth about who you are, you will never lose yourself again, no matter whether you gain weight or lose weight.

PART TWO:
DIET AND SELF-RECONSTRUCTION

(The Putting Together of Self and Diet)

CHAPTER 8 :

CHANGING YOUR BELIEFS ABOUT YOUR SELF-WORTH

STAGE #1:
THE HEALING POWER OF SELF-FORGIVENESS

The first rock bottom question you need to learn the truth about is, "Why can't I lose weight?" In actual fact, the question should be, "Why can't you maintain your weight loss?" As you have learned, you have lost lots of weight; you have just not been able to keep it off.

By going through the four-stage diet cycle of self-destruction and learning why the diet approach does not work, you will have answered your first rock bottom question. By using the rational and critical thinking powers of your mind, you should have proven to yourself without a shadow of a doubt that the perfect, fast, and easy diet approach to weight loss is why you failed and that it was not your fault. Which means there was nothing inherently wrong with you; it was the approach you were using. Once you believe this, you can finally forgive yourself. Forgiving yourself is the first stage in the healing process.

Forgiving yourself for failing because it was not your fault begins the process of healing and repairing your relationship with yourself and the world. When you forgive yourself you can start moving forward instead of holding on to your past mistakes. This means you can stop dwelling on how much of a failure you are, which allows you to start letting go of some of the toxic G.A.A.S.S. you have been holding on to.

Just like when you have a fight with a friend and are mad at each other, only when you forgive each other can you heal the hurt and move on with your relationship. Forgiving yourself brings some peace within and makes you feel better about yourself. It replaces some of your negative and depressive feelings with positive and happy feelings. As the poet and author William Arthur Ward said, "Forgiveness is a funny thing, it warms the heart and cools the sting."

Besides the benefit of being able to forgive yourself, when you no longer believe that the perfect, fast, and easy diet approach to weight loss works, you will also stop using it. When you stop using this approach, you stop the cycle of self-destruction you have been trapped in. As a result, you break your dependency on following such diets to achieve weight loss success.

Once you know the truth about the perfect, fast, and easy diet approach and have forgiven yourself, you can move on to changing the false, destructive beliefs you have developed about yourself and life.

CHANGING YOUR BELIEFS ABOUT WHO YOU ARE

The next rock bottom question to answer is, "Who am I?" As discussed, when you regain the weight you lost, you believe you are worthless, powerless, hopeless, and cursed. You believe you're not worthy enough as you are because you're bigger than ever and you believe you're powerless, hopeless, and cursed because you have regained back all your weight plus more, despite trying your best. As a result, you no longer accept, love, or believe in yourself.

It's these false self-beliefs you have developed as a result of failing to lose weight that you have to change if you want to stop yourself from gaining weight and losing yourself. As the O.D.G. (original diet guru) Richard Simmons said during a television interview, "The only way in all the years and the millions of people that I've helped, the only way is number one: like yourself." He also stated to do two more things, which was to watch your portions and to move. This is why it's so important to learn the truth about yourself, eating healthy, and exercising. If you want to be inspired to love yourself, check him out online.

Let's first investigate the belief that you are not worthy enough because you are overweight.

YOU ARE NOT YOUR BODY IMAGE

Due to following diets, a large part (if not all) of your self-worth became dependent on your body image. As you learned, when you started to regain your lost weight, you now had to lose weight to feel good about yourself and as a result, your body image became who you are. You only feel good about yourself if you look a certain way, weigh a certain amount, and wear a certain size.

You have to ask yourself, "Is your physical appearance who you are and where true self-worth comes from? Are you your stomach, your arms, your thighs, or your ass? Are you how much you weigh or what size you are?" Yes, you do have a face and body that you see, use, and are judged by on a daily basis, but that doesn't mean they're the most important parts of who you are—not by a long shot.

All of your focus has been on striving to achieve the perfect body image so you can be acceptable, worthy, and powerful. It's all you valued about who you are. Again, this is because you believed the hype that if you look good, you will feel good and your life will be good.

Even though you see and hear those diet ads every day telling you to change your body, it's not what you need to change. You are not your body, you just think you are and that's the problem. You have to learn that your looks and body size (which as you know you can lose and gain) does not determine if you feel good or if your life is good—your thinking does. As Dr. David D. Burns, M.D. said in his bestseller *Feeling Good*, "You feel the way you do right now because of the thoughts you are thinking at this moment."[36]

As stated earlier, before you can change your weight, you have to change your mind. This is because you are your mind, not your weight. You spent all that time trying to change and develop your body to improve yourself and life, when you should have been focused on trying to change and develop your mind.

YOU ARE YOUR MIND

Although it's not seen, your inner mind is the most important and valuable part of yourself. The mind is where you are and is where you find your true self. Your true self is found in your higher thinking. As the philosopher Descartes said, "I think, therefore I am," and as martial arts legend Bruce Lee said, "as you think, so shall you become." You are, in other words, who you think you are. This is why to change who you are, you have to change your thinking.

You are a self-concept, an idea, a description, that can be changed. The words and labels you use to describe yourself can be reversed. Who you are is not set in stone or decided by fate; it's decided by your mind and what you think about yourself.

Your belief that you are unworthy, powerless, and cursed,

because it's part of your DNA is false. It's all in your head. Your entire selfhood and world is in your mind. Your beliefs about yourself and the world becomes your reality. If you want to change how you see yourself and the world, all you have to do is change your perspective.

INCREASING YOUR SELF-UNDERSTANDING

By following and failing at diet programs, you developed a closed, narrow, and distorted view about yourself and the world you live in. Your view of yourself and life can be as small as the neighborhood you grew up in or encompass the whole universe and beyond. The only limit is the one you put on yourself.

Your mind's ability to expand its knowledge and language is limitless. You may not be able to change some of your physical characteristics, but you can change the amount you know. As the scientist Albert Einstein stated, "A mind that is open to a new idea changes sizes." In other words, the more you know, the more you grow.

The more you learn and know about your identity and reality, the bigger your self-concept becomes. By rationally and critically studying yourself and other subjects like anthropology, astronomy, biology, history, philosophy, psychology, religion, sociology, and spirituality, along with learning from other cultures and other people's experiences, you will gain a greater understanding about who you truly are. You will go from a small self-understanding to a very large self-understanding. Your perspective on how you see yourself and life will change.

It was this truth that you have the power to change who you are by changing your thinking that changed my life. I always thought I was who I was. I always thought I was my name, my face, my body, my weight, my nationality, my race(s), and my address. I never thought you could change who you are. This was because I never knew I was my thinking. The poet and philosopher Henry David Thoreau articulated this truth when he wrote, "Thought is the sculptor who can create the person you want to be."

I never thought about my inner or universal self. I never thought there was more to me than my outer physical self. I only focused on the external parts of me I (and others) could see and never thought about any other parts of me. My mind and my thinking is something I most definitely did not think about or pay any attention to.

That was until I learned that my thinking about myself was both the problem and the solution.

Learning and finding out the truth that you are more than you think you are is captured in the play *Our Town* written by novelist and American playwright Thorton Wilder. On an envelope addressed to one of the characters it included the usual name, county/city, and country, but also included Continent of North America, Western Hemisphere, the Earth, the Solar System, the Universe, and the Mind of God. Until you use your higher thinking powers to learn and expand the truth about who you are, you will remain trapped in your own limited, negative, and false thinking.

YOU ARE WORTHY

I'm going to share with you what I learned about myself using my rational and critical thinking powers to search for who I am. What I learned is the universal truth that every person who searches for the truth about themselves discovers—that your true self-worth, power, hope, and happiness is found within yourself, not outside of yourself.

Everything you have been searching for is within you. When you use the powers of your mind to search for the truth about who you are, you will learn the self-evident truths that you are worthy, powerful, and blessed. This is what will change your false beliefs and thinking about who you are and who you need to be.

Let's first take a look at all the truths that make you a worthy person.

YOU ARE EARTH

You are worthy just for being here today on this planet. You are part of and connected to this amazing and spectacular place. The Power(s) that created this planet also created you. From the beautiful blue sky, to the majestic mountains, to the luscious landscapes, to the towering trees, to the roaring rivers, to the setting sun, to any amazing animal or insect you can think of, you share the same Creator. This makes you amazing and spectacular.

We are all interrelated and interdependent on Earth. For example, like Earth, Humans are mostly made up of water and need it for life. We also breathe the Earth's air and eat its food and use its other natural resources for life. As Inuit author Sheila Watt-Cloutier stated,

"We are an extension of the land, we are the land and the land is us."[37]

Everything created here is inherently worthy. We are all children of creation. Just being in and part of nature: seeing its beauty, hearing its sounds, smelling its fragrances, touching its textures, and feeling its wind—makes you feel worthy. Being worthy is your birth-right.

YOU ARE SPECIAL

Just like everything else in nature, humans are a diverse species that come in all shapes, shades, and sizes. What a boring and bland world this would be if everybody and everything were all the same. Humans like, and are stimulated by, seeing contrast and things that are different. As it is said, variety is the spice of life.

You live in a world that is awe-inspiring, interesting, and oh-so-beautiful because of all the diversity that exists. Just look at the variety of faces, fruits, flowers, flavors, and furry creatures there are. It's pleasing to both the senses and the mind.

The one version of beauty and power that you see in main-stream media doesn't represent the true complexity and diversity of our species. For example, you rarely if ever, see an "overweight" person or a person in a wheelchair as the romantic lead in any movie or television show, nor on the cover of any magazine. These opportunities are usu-ally reserved for people who possess the so-called perfect body image.

Whenever you are amongst a group of people or are walking down the street, look around and you will see that we all look different and we all look the same. We all have some of the same features and we have some different ones. What is the same is we all have features that we like and some that we don't. The funny thing is that when you put us all together we create the perfect picture. This is why diversity should be celebrated and promoted.

Everybody is everybody. There is no one type that is better than the other. No matter how you were born, you have something different and special to offer. You have your own particular strengths, talents, and ways of seeing the world that is different from any other person on Earth. Embrace your uniqueness. Don't try to be anybody or anything else other than yourself. This sentiment was expressed brilliantly by columnist Chuck Gallozzi: "In a world of perfect people, everyone is the same. Everyone is plastic, molded after perfection. Everyone is lifeless. But in the real world, people have imperfections, weaknesses, and vulnerabilities. This is what defines people. It gives them personality. It also gives them the opportunity to display great strength and courage by acting despite their fears."[38]

Put more simply by popular children's TV host Mister Rogers, "everybody is so special because everybody is different."

YOU ARE PRICELESS

There are billions of people on this planet but only one of you. When people say, you are one in a million, they are selling you short. Two people from all the billions of people had to come together to make you a possibility. Out of the thousands of sperm and hundreds of eggs, you were made. You are a miracle of life.

There will never again be another you. You are one of a kind, a rare jewel. Your voice, laugh, smile, size, sensibilities, fingerprints, and even heartbeat are all unique to you. You are your own masterpiece.

YOU ARE A PHENOMENON

You are a biological marvel. You have eyes that see, ears that hear, a tongue that tastes, a nose that smells, and an entire body that senses touch. You have a heart that beats, kidneys that purify, and an immune system that heals. You are like the Marvel comic/movie superhero Wolverine, in the sense that you too can heal from illnesses, cuts, and wounds.

You have a skeletal system that is comprised of 206 bones. As well, you have a respiratory system with lungs that breathe 18,000 to 20,000 breaths a day. There is also the muscular, digestive, and nervous systems, along with many other systems that do complicated and important jobs.

Most impressive of all is your brain. The brain is often compared to a super computer. Approximately ninety percent of the 10 billion neurons (nerve cells) in your body are found in the brain.[39] You are always connected to your neural networks that contain the files that hold the different knowledge and skills you have. Your brain has a limitless capacity to build new networks which allows you to continuously program yourself with new knowledge and skills.

Your brain can process and store vast amounts of data collected from your senses and experiences. It can also organize and analyze this information and make predictions and decisions about what the best answer or action to take is. It's been said the brain, on average, makes 35,000 decisions a day.

You also have a built-in GPS system that can create a mental map of your surroundings and direct you to your destination.

You don't have to know how everything works to know you are a remarkable creation. Joel Thuna, who knows how the heart works said this: "Your heart is an amazing organ. It continuously pumps oxygen and nutrient-rich blood throughout your body. This powerhouse beats 100,000 times per day, pumping five or six quarts of blood each minute or about 8000 litres each day. At rest, a normal heart beats around 50 to 99 times a minute. Exercise, emotions, fever, and medications can cause your heart to beat faster, sometimes to well over 100 beats per minute."[40]

YOU ARE A STAR

You are also a universal being. You live on Earth, which is spinning around the sun at the rate of 100,000 km/hour. The planet Earth is in space and is part of the galaxy known as the Milky Way. The Milky Way is part of billions of other galaxies.

When you look up and see all those stars in the night sky you are looking at yourself. The same chemical elements that make up the stars above is also what you are made of. That makes you a star. As the scientist Carl Sagan said, "We are all made up of star stuff."

Every now and then take a look upward and remind yourself that you are on a planet that is rotating and revolving in a universe filled with other galaxies, planets, and stars. This will help you focus on who you truly are.

KNOWING YOUR TRUE WORTH

Once you have learned for yourself what makes you worthy, how you think about yourself will change. Due to gaining a deeper understanding about yourself, you will now focus on other more important parts of who you are, instead of just focusing on your body image. Your mind will now be filled with positive thoughts about your identity, which in turn, will fill you with positive feelings about who you are.

The knowledge you learn about why you are worthy becomes the language/words you use to describe and think about yourself.

Before when you told yourself you were unworthy because you were overweight, you had no rational arguments to fight back with. Now you do.

STAGE #2: THE HEALING POWER OF SELF-ACCEPTANCE AND SELF-LOVE

Accepting and loving yourself for who you are because of who you are, is the second step in healing yourself. When you believe you are okay and are worthy just for being you, your feelings of worthlessness and toxic shame are replaced with feelings of self-worth and pride. You no longer reject and dislike yourself, but instead accept and love yourself.

It's the self-acceptance and self-love that allows you to heal from the depression and pain of self-rejection and self-hate due to being overweight. Your mind will no longer be focused on and worried about how much you weigh, but rather on how worthy you are. This helps to resolve your identity-conflict and bring peace within yourself. You will no longer be fighting and hurting yourself, but will instead love, encourage, and take care of yourself. There is no more ideal self, only the real (worthy) self remains.

Knowing the truth about who you are is where true feelings of self-worth come from, not from how you look. When you feel good about who you are and love yourself, you are motivated to do the best for yourself. You will no longer want to lose weight because you dislike yourself, but because you love yourself.

When you truly accept and love yourself, you break your dependency on having to achieve the perfect body image to feel good about yourself. Having the perfect body image is no longer a value-priority you have to achieve to feel worthy. You accept and love yourself unconditionally because of who you are.

There was a British show on television called *"How To Look Good Naked"* hosted by stylist Gok Wan that helped women realize they had a distorted body image and were unnecessarily hating and shaming themselves. He would tell the women that they were beautiful the way they were, and that self-confidence is what makes you sexy. Then he would show them what clothes and hairstyle to wear to make them look their best right now, not when they lose weight. There were no messages about changing who you are, but rather accepting and loving yourself and the body you're in. As Gok Wan stated, he wanted to "reawaken their inner goddess."

SELF-AFFIRMATIONS

To facilitate the process of accepting and loving yourself, reflect daily on the reasons why you are worthy. Every day you wake up tell yourself how worthy you are. Stand in front of the mirror, look yourself in the eyes, and tell yourself over and over again why you are worthy. For example, you could say to yourself, I am worthy because:

- "I am Earth."
- "I am priceless."
- "I am a super being."
- "I am one of a kind."
- "I am a super star."

In a self-help skit on the comedy show Saturday Night Live called "Daily Affirmations With Stuart Smalley" (it's on YouTube if you want to view it) he would look in the mirror and tell himself:

- "I deserve good things."
- "I'm entitled to my share of happiness."
- "I refuse to beat myself up."
- "I am an attractive person."
- "I am fun to be with."

Every time you say these positive self-affirmations to yourself it makes you feel good about who you are. I've heard it said many times by psychologists that seventy to eighty percent of your internal self-talk is negative. As well, when you are in a state of depression, your false, destructive beliefs repeat over and over in your head. This is why you want to say positive self-affirmations to yourself every day, all day. Author of *Minding the Body, Mending the Mind* Joan Borysenko, Ph.D., put it like this: "The use of affirmation gradually erodes old ingrained patterns of thinking, substituting a new understanding and fresh frame of reference."[41]

Once you have proved to yourself you are inherently worthy, you now have to learn what makes you inherently powerful.

CHAPTER 9:

CHANGING YOUR BELIEFS ABOUT YOUR SELF-POWER

As previously mentioned, due to not being able to stop yourself from regaining all your weight back after trying you're best, you have little confidence or hope that you can be successful and happy. You tell yourself that you're a failure and that you can't, won't, and will never lose weight. You believe you have been cursed to this fate by the powers that be and are powerless to change your situation. As a result, you quit on yourself and no longer try to diet. These are the thoughts that are causing you to feel helpless, hopeless, and depressed, and it's these feelings that drive you to overeat and gain more weight than ever.

Since you have already learned that it's not your fault for failing, this means that you're not a failure or powerless. By using an approach that doesn't work you were set up to fail. This is why you were not successful, not because there was something inherently wrong with you. Again, you have to learn the truth about yourself and learn just how inherently powerful you are. You have to use your rational and critical thinking powers to learn the truth that you are a born:

FIGHTER

All humans are born with the fighting spirit and the instinct to survive. The story of the underdog, winning against insurmountable odds, like David versus Goliath in the Bible, is a core part of the human psyche. Most people cheer for the "underdog," because they see themselves as the "little person" having to fight powerful, bigger forces to survive.

Just to survive as a species here on Earth, humans had to fight environmental disasters, diseases, and killer creatures. Every day, to some degree, is a fight for survival. You have to fight just to make ends meet. Some people like boxers, literally do. If you are alive, that proves you are a fighter.

There are a lot of challenges, conflicts, and crises in life. Failing and having to pick yourself back up after losses or sickness is a part of life. Everybody feels like giving up at times. It all can feel like too much to deal with. You have to fight with yourself to not give into those feelings.

The fact that you were ever able to be successful at all using diet programs should be proof enough that you are powerful. Against all odds, you fought and picked yourself back up day after day, month after month, year after year until you finally achieved success. You're a fighter and a winner, not a quitter and a failure. You have proved that you are resilient and can persevere. Stop telling yourself lies. See yourself for who you truly are.

The truth is, the only time you ever fail is when you don't try or quit. There is no success without failure. As the saying goes, "winners never quit and quitters never win." For example, there was a baseball pitcher in the major leagues who lost for three years until he finally won a game. The winning of that one game is not what's important—it's the fact that he did not quit over all those years of losing. It shows you how much he believed in himself despite the doubt that must have been there from within and without (teammates, coaches, fans, announcers). He persevered and persisted through a difficult situation—this is what makes him a winner.

Reflect on your life and think about all the times you have picked yourself back up after a tough loss and overcame the odds. Don't let what happened to you following diets distort who you really are.

ACHIEVER

You have a history of being successful and achieving your goals. Ever since you were born, you have been achieving milestones and passing tests. It's important to recognize and acknowledge your accomplishments. You have to believe and know that you have the power to achieve the goal of managing your weight. The proof is there.

Whether learning new knowledge or a new skill, graduating from school, gaining employment, winning a ribbon/trophy, or checking off a to-do-list, use your mind to reflect on your life and go over all your achievements (big and small). Writer them all down and you might be surprised how big the list is. You wouldn't be where you are today if you were not an achiever.

You can achieve any goal as long as you break it down into small, manageable parts. Setting a goal of losing fifty pounds can be overwhelming, but if you break it down to losing one pound a week, so you can lose four pounds a month over twelve months, it seems doable.

A lot of businesses use the S.M.A.R.T. acronym, to ensure their company goals can be achieved. By using the S.M.A.R.T. approach you can ensure that your goal is: Specific, Measurable, Attainable, Realistic, and Timely. This S.M.A.R.T. approach to achieving goals is definitely not used by the perfect, fast, and easy diet approach.

CREATOR

You were created by and are part of whoever or whatever you believe created this magnificent world and the universe beyond. Due to your powerful brain, you also have been given the power to create. Research in the last 45 years has shown that each person is born with creative ability.[42] Remember back to when you were a child and expressed your creativity through play, drawings, dancing, and paintings.

For the most part, you have the power to create your own identity and your own life. For example, someone who wants to become a doctor will take science courses, volunteer at a hospital, and study to achieve good grades. They do this so they will be accepted into a good medical school. They know this is the path that will help them create the life they envisioned for themselves. As writer Chuck Gallozzi's said, "Without a map, or vision, we cannot predict our future, but with a map, we become seers. We can see into the future because we knowingly create it."[43]

Whether it's a career or even what you're going to do this weekend, you have a vision in your head that you want to turn into reality. It's through visions that a lot of people create the life they want. Life is like a blank canvass where you can paint the picture of the life you want. You are the artist of your own life, the director of your own movie, and the author of your own story. Why not make yourself a superhero and live a super life?

Through your thoughts and actions you have the power to create the type of day you want and the type of life you want to live. This includes creating your own healthy eating and living plan. You were born with the power to turn your dreams into reality. Look inside your mind and either write, paint, or draw your inner visions when you see them. Then fight to stick to your vision.

LEARNER

You were born with the most powerful brain of all the species on the planet. You are an intelligent and thinking being. The word Homo sapiens means "man the wise."[44] You were built to learn.

Through every sense you have, your mind processes and learns from the information it gathers. You learn from what you see, smell, hear, touch, taste and of course, from what you think and feel. You learn from every interaction and experience in your environment. From every word you read, to every person you see, speak and listen to—all the information you learn about yourself, others, and the world is stored in your brain's memory. Your memory, along with the amount you can learn, is limitless.

Your brain is constantly assessing, evaluating, and analyzing your environment and experiences so it can figure out who you are (strengths and weaknesses) and how to live to survive and be happy. This is why you ask the who, what, where, when, why, and how questions. Your brain is like the *Enquirer* tabloid—it wants and needs to know.

All of the learning and education you have been receiving since you were a baby was done with the aim of turning you into an independent, successful, and mature adult. From crawling and walking, to potty training and brushing your teeth, to eating and speaking, to reading and writing, to basic math and budgeting, to learning social rules and how to drive, you have been learning knowledge and developing skills for a long time. With patience, practice, persistence, and passion, you can learn almost any knowledge and develop any skill or behaviour.

If you have passed grades/graduated from school and/or have learned life and job skills, you have to know and believe you have the power to learn how to eat and not to eat in order to be healthy. You have been using different diet programs for a long time. You have acquired a lot of knowledge and skills to know what works for you and what doesn't. You can use this information to develop your own eating program.

Chances are you have more knowledge and experience than most of the people that are telling you they have the answer. By the slim chance you don't, you do have the ability to read books/magazines/web pages, listen to radio shows/podcasts, and watch television programs to acquire knowledge on the topics of nutrition and exercise.

We are living in the information age and knowledge about everything and anything is everywhere.

SELF-REGULATOR

You are a conscious being, and as such you have the power of self-awareness. Not only are you aware of your outer self and surroundings, you are also aware of your inner mind and body. This is what gives you the power to control and change the thoughts and evaluations in your mind and as a result, your emotions and behaviour.

It cannot be said enough, the most important truth you need to learn about yourself is that it's the beliefs, thoughts, and evaluations in your mind that create the feelings that drive you to act the way you do. This is why your attention needs to be focused on what is going on inside your mind and body. You need to be aware of what you're feeling in your body and saying in your mind if you want to be able to control and change your feelings and behaviour.

The only thing you truly have some control over is how you think, feel, and behave. You cannot control how somebody else thinks, feels, or behaves, or how life behaves—all you can control is how you think, feel, and behave. For example, if someone calls you a negative name, your natural reaction is to be upset or angry and to run away or call the person a name back. Now you are acting emotionally and are in a bad or sad mood.

You have to ask yourself who has the power. Does another person have the power to make you react negatively or do you have the power to control how you feel and behave? Given your power to be aware of your internal reactions and your power to choose how you think, feel, and behave, you have the power to change your emotional reaction and can instead choose to laugh or say nothing. This is what gives humans the power of free will, and it is why each person is held responsible for their own behaviour.

It's takes effort, but we have the ability to control our natural and conditioned emotional reactions, and can consciously choose how we think, feel, and act. No external person or no external object like food, has power over us. As the former first lady Eleanor Roosevelt said, "No one can make you feel inferior without your consent." All that matters is what you think. If you don't think you're inferior then you're not, no matter what anyone else says.

Gallozzi also powerfully said, "we cannot make any real

progress until we admit to ourselves, only I can hold myself back. Only I can stand in my own way. Only I can help myself. Only I can take personal responsibility. Only I can transform myself from a victim of circumstances to a reasoning, choice-making, action oriented person. Only I can make the decision to stop acting like a victim and start taking charge of my life."[45]

By controlling your inner mind and body, you have the power to control your destructive emotional reactions and destructive emotional behaviours, which you have to be able to do to not only to control your eating, but also to live in society. Every day in order to survive in the world, you have to be able to control yourself. If not, you would be reading this book from jail and would have no job. Many of us have impulses to yell or hit someone when upset, but we know we can't because it's not the right thing to do and we know it will lead to negative consequences.

As well, to be successful at school, work, and home, we have to be able to control our emotions and impulses in order to complete tasks we don't feel like or hate doing. For example, when having to learn a new job at work or a new math equation at school, you make lots of mistakes and become frustrated and impatient and want to quit. You have to rationally tell yourself that it takes time to learn anything new and that with practice you will improve.

Our rational and critical mind is the only tool we have at our disposal that has the power to control our natural and conditioned emotional reactions and urges. Our feelings and urges are strong, but our conscious, rational mind is even stronger. We have the power to make ourselves act how we want, when we want. You can clearly control yourself, so you are powerful enough to control your emotional eating and are not helpless and hopeless.

PROBLEM-SOLVER

By using your higher thinking powers, you have the ability to solve most problems you encounter. Problems like people come in all sizes. Some are small and can be solved quickly, while others are big and require time and work. Figuring out how to land on the moon was a big problem; figuring out why your internet connection is not working is a small problem.

Problems can be solved by thinking logically and/or by thinking outside of the box. You can also try different strategies to solve a problem. For example, you can brainstorm to come up with as many solutions as you can and can then use your analytical and evaluative powers to pick the best one(s). You can then try it out to see if it works. If it doesn't, you try the next best one and so on, until you find a solution that works. As long as you're trying to solve the problem instead of avoiding or escaping it, you are on the right track.

You can also do research, read books, go to a professional, use a search engine, ask and listen to family and friends, but in the end, you have to use your own mind to figure out what solution will work for you. For example, for people trying to quit smoking, the patch might work for one person, while therapy or hypnosis might work for another.

Your brain is so good at solving problems it does it even while you're doing something else. This is known as the "Eureka Phenomenon." The story goes that Sir Isaac Newton was sitting under a tree relaxing and an apple fell and hit him on the head and in that moment he discovered the answer to the gravity problem he had been working on and cried, "Eureka." This is why when you are having difficulty finding a solution to a problem, the best thing you can do is go do something else in hopes that the answer will come to you in a flash of insight.

You have been solving problems for a long time, whether they be school, peer, family, personal, financial, or work problems. You have even solved problems for fun. Think puzzles, crosswords, and the Rubik's Cube. Reflect on the problems you have confronted and solved in your lifetime. You have all the powers you need to solve your problem of why you can't manage your weight.

STAGE #3: THE HEALING POWER OF SELF-BELIEF

Believing in yourself because you know who you are and know how powerful you are is the next step in the healing process. When you believe you are powerful and that you have the power to make yourself successful and happy, your feelings of helplessness and hopelessness are changed into feelings of confidence and hope.

When you have learned for yourself that you have the power to control how you think, feel, and act by controlling your mind and body, your focus changes. You will no longer focus on your external body image/appearance to give you power—instead, you will focus on your internal mind/body. You know by doing so, you can make yourself feel good and do good.

It's a powerful feeling to know that you can control yourself and can get yourself to feel and act the way you want to. When you know you have the power to control yourself, your locus of control permanently changes from external to internal. This is when you truly become a self-empowered and independent person.

This knowledge of your self-power gives you the confidence and hope that you will be successful and happy even when you face challenges and disappointment. As you know, if you have no self-belief and hope you have no motivation to even try. This is when you hear the dreaded and self-defeating "can't" word.

When you believe you can't, you paralyze yourself. The anxiety, insecurity, and fear that is created by having this belief prevents you from being able to act competently or act at all. You fail before you even try.

To doubt oneself is natural. When you're trying to achieve a goal or a dream, you don't know for sure if you can or will do it until you do. As well, because frustration and making mistakes is part of the learning and goal-achieving process, you will want to give up and quit. To continue on day after day, month after month, year after year, and not quit, you have to believe in yourself and know you will eventually succeed. For those of you old enough to remember the story, to achieve anything you have to be like the little engine that could and think you can. Better still is telling yourself you know you can.

It's this self-belief that will not only carry you through the healing and rebuilding process, but is what will also carry you through all the tough times when you want to give in to the negativity and pain and quit. Every day you have to say positive self-affirmations and remind yourself that you are powerful because you're a born:

- Fighter.

- Achiever.

- Creator.

- Learner.

- Self-Regulator.

- Problem-Solver.

Since you now know that you are inherently powerful and

feel powerful, you are ready to learn the truth about your life and how blessed you are. When you learn this truth about your life, you will change how you see your life.

CHAPTER 10:

CHANGING YOUR BELIEFS ABOUT YOUR LIFE

REALITY CHECK

The final rock bottom self-belief you need to change is your belief that your life is not great because you are overweight and your belief that you've been cursed to this fate by your Creator. Since you are bigger than ever and are feeling pain and depression, you dislike this aspect of yourself and life and are mad at your Creator. All you can focus on is the weight you gained and how unhappy you are about it.

You feel it's not fair that this has happened to you. You have the "woe is me blues." After an epic disappointment, it's a natural response to be upset and feel sorry for yourself. The danger comes when you do it for too long.

When you're in pain and feeling depressed, it's hard to see the light amidst the darkness. All you can see is the negative and the bad. While in the rock bottom stage, you look at your life based on what you don't have, instead of what you do have. You are so focused on the weight and the pain that you don't pay any attention to all of the good things about yourself and life or how much worse it could be.

You have to be able to put yourself and your life into its proper, rational perspective, especially when things go wrong. No one is perfect and no one's life is perfect. We all have our cross to bear. If you look rationally and critically at the facts of life, there are good times and bad times, victories and losses. No person wins forever or never experiences struggle and disappointment.

Now I know from first-hand experience that regaining more weight than ever is a very painful experience, but when you think objectively about yourself and your life, you will learn that it's not the worst thing in the world. In fact, when you use the powers of your mind to think about the world you live in, you will learn that you have not been cursed by your Creator, but in fact, have been blessed.

When you look at life realistically, you see that some people are born with parents, some with one, and some with none. Others are born with no sight, no hearing, no arms, no legs, no hands, no fingers, and some people lose these body parts by accident. Some people are born poor, some rich, and some in-between. As it states in the Bible, "By the grace of God go I."

If you have your fingers, your hands, arms, mobility, sight, and hearing, you are lucky. If you are safe and have shelter, food, and a decent job, you are very, very lucky. When people bless their food, they are giving thanks that the family has food for today because there are other people who have no food and maybe tomorrow it's us.

Millions on this planet are not safe, do not have a place to live or enough to eat, and have no means or hope of being able to do so. It won't take long for you to think of some places in your own country or around the world where people are living in sub-standard or war-torn conditions. You have to thank your lucky stars if you are not.

If you want to be alive, you are blessed. The truth is, you could perish today. As the wise say, tomorrow is not promised. Accidents and bad things happen to thousands of good people every day.

The daily news is filled with stories of people being harmed or dying unexpectedly. Whether it's trains, planes, or automobiles, accidents happen. As well, there are people, including children, who are diagnosed with terminal illnesses on a daily basis. It's brutal and devastatingly sad, but that is reality and it's important to be aware of it so you can put yourself and your life into its proper perspective.

This is what the Canadian hero Terry Fox, who was diagnosed with cancer in his early twenties and lost his leg, was inspirationally able to do. Instead of letting the "woe is me blues" consume him, he thought about all the children he saw in the hospital battling cancer and decided to raise money for cancer research by running across Canada. Although he passed away before completing his run, Terry Fox raised over 24 million dollars and since then his foundation has raised over 600 hundred million and counting.

There was an article in the newspaper entitled "Awareness Of Death Makes Life More Precious," that discussed the importance of not trying to deny your fragility but to instead embrace it.[46] By doing so, you learn to appreciate and be happy with the life you have right now, even with all the problems you might be facing. You realize as long as you and your loved ones are alive and well, there really are no major problems. So, while you have it, enjoy your life.

The writer of the article Abdul-Rehman Malik used a quote

by the Prophet Muhammad to highlight the importance of appreciating all the blessings in your life while you have them: "Take advantage of five things before five others occur: your youth before your old age, your health before your sickness, your wealth before your poverty, your leisure before your work and your life before your death."

If you are not thankful for these things while you have them, you can't help but be disappointed and regretful when you no longer have them. It reinforces the belief to not take any blessing for granted. You have to try your best to appreciate each day and moment you have been given because it could be your last.

After learning the facts of life, you will prove to yourself that you have a blessed life and are not cursed. This truth forces you to focus on all the good things in your life rather than on the few bad things. This makes you appreciate yourself, your family, your friends, your life, and your Creator, which in turn makes you feel positive rather than negative.

STAGE #4: THE HEALING POWER OF GRATITUDE

Showing gratitude and knowing how blessed you are, is the last stage of the healing process. When you believe you are blessed, it changes how you think and live. You're past disappointments and grievances with your life and Creator will be resolved. You will no longer feel depressed but will be thankful and will feel contentment and peace with who you are and your place in the world/universe.

You will also start to appreciate not only all that you have, but will also start to appreciate the moment and the day you have been given. You take nothing for granted because you know it can be taken away from you at any time. This is how you learn to focus your attention on just "being in the moment" without thinking about past failures or future "doom and gloom." You're just grateful for being alive at this very moment in time.

When you know the truth about life, your problem of being overweight starts to seem small compared to someone who is going through true life and death hardships. Rather than focusing on being overweight, more of your attention is focused on all the blessings in your life. You find yourself dwelling on the positive instead of the negative. With each blessed thought, you can't help but smile and feel good. As author Marianne Williamson said, "Joy is what happens to us when we allow ourselves to recognize how good things really are."

Every time you count your blessings instead of focusing on the negative, you are refilling yourself with joy, strength, passion, peace, and hope. It's these feelings that give you the strength to continue to fight the good fight like eating healthy. This is why you want to remain focused on your blessings on a full-time basis.

Even during true tough times, you learn that you still have blessings to count. By doing this, it prevents you from going all the way down. Spending some time counting your blessings gives you a break from your problems and gives you something to feel good about.

When you're feeling pain or are stressed and depressed, you are triggered emotionally to want to eat unhealthy to escape. You have to learn for yourself that there is no better coping mechanism for stress, negativity, and pain, than being grateful for all you have. This is how you will learn the secret, that managing your weight is more about COUNTING YOUR BLESSINGS THAN COUNTING CALORIES.

PRACTICING GRATEFULNESS

An exercise that can help you maintain a state of gratefulness is to write down five to ten things you are grateful for (e.g., life, family, health, job, etcetera) and whenever you are dealing with a challenge or upset and are feeling sorry for yourself, repeat your list to yourself and think about all the people in the world who have it worse than you. You can also remind yourself of the Persian proverb: I cried because I had no shoes until I saw someone with no feet.

A lot of religious people sing hymns to help remind themselves to be grateful. A good example of a classic hymn religious people use is, "Count your many blessings, name them one by one, and it will surprise you what the Lord has done."

If you're not religious and don't have a hymn to sing, you could pick a song that you know gives you positive and hopeful feelings. As long as you are focused on your blessings and singing on the inside, nothing can take away your joy. This is why they tell you to "whistle while you work."

Whistling and singing are more powerful than words because they trigger a stronger, positive emotional reaction within you. Even if you don't like your job, as long as you have joy in your heart and are grateful for at least having a job and being alive, you will remain positive.

As well, at least once a day try to take a moment to be aware of the blessing that you are alive. Take a look around at all the beauty and give thanks. Stay in the moment and mediate on this. The goal is to reach the point where you permanently meditate on your blessings and live the daily moments of your life in full joy and appreciation. Even, and especially, during the down times.

NEW SELF-BELIEF SYSTEM

After using the rational and critical thinking powers of your mind to prove to yourself that the rock bottom beliefs you developed about yourself and your life are false, you will be ready to adopt the beliefs you learned are true. These new, true, rational beliefs form your new self-understanding. As a result, you now believe you are acceptable, worthy, powerful, and blessed. This becomes your new answer to your rock bottom question, "who am I?"

When your mind is focused on your new, true, rational self-beliefs, your negative and painful emotions of worthlessness, powerlessness, and hopelessness that make you feel stressed and depressed and trigger you to binge to escape, are replaced with feelings of worth, power, gratefulness, hope, and happiness. You feel better about yourself and life, which in turn energizes and motivates you to want to do good things for yourself like eat healthy and exercise.

In order to facilitate the healing and rebuilding process, you have to meditate on and repeat your true beliefs to yourself everyday. Your false beliefs and negative feelings are strong (especially if you're depressed), and it takes time and daily repeating of the truth for your rational beliefs to take over your mind and for your positive feelings to take over your body. You have to repeat to yourself over and over that:

- You believe it's not your fault that you weigh more than ever and you forgive yourself.

- You believe you are worthy just the way you are and accept and love yourself.

- You believe you are powerful and can and will learn to manage your weight.

- You believe you are blessed.

Once you have used your higher thinking powers to learn the truth about the diet approach, yourself, and reality, the next rock bottom question to answer is,"How can I lose weight?" Until you learned the truth, your answer was to follow the perfect, fast, and easy diet approach. Since you no longer believe in this answer and now believe in yourself, it's time to try a new approach to losing and managing your weight. Before you can do this, you first have to change the false beliefs you have developed about eating healthy and exercising.

CHAPTER 11

CHANGING YOUR FALSE BELIEFS ABOUT EATING HEALTHY

FALSE BELIEF #1: EATING HEALTHY MEANS STARVING YOURSELF

By listening to and following fad diet programs, you believe that to lose weight you have to restrict calories and eat as little food as you can. You end up believing that if you're not starving yourself, you're not eating healthy.

There was one diet program I was on in my mid-teens that told me to eat 690 calories. That is far less than half the calories I should have been eating to not only fulfill my nutritional requirements, but also to lose weight.*

Eating too few calories not only depletes you of the energy you need to eat healthy and exercise, but it also makes losing weight harder. When you drastically restrict your calories, it triggers a starvation response. This slows down your metabolism and makes your body conserve the fat you have. Fat has the most calories in it, so that is what's preserved.

As well, when you don't eat enough your blood sugar level drops, and as a result you feel tired and will be triggered to refuel yourself by eating a lot. Your mind and body needs the correct amount of food throughout the day in order to function properly. If you eat too little or too much, you will experience negative effects. For example, a headache or dizziness.

These extreme, restrictive diets for some people can lead to eating disorders, such as bulimia and anorexia. I have both purged and used fasting in an attempt to lose weight. Luckily, neither developed into an eating disorder. Think back to your own restrictive diet history of starving yourself or using other dangerous methods to lose weight.

---

*   *At the back of this book in Appendix 1(a) and 1(b), you will find information about calories.*

As you learned, food restriction is also what causes the value-conflict within yourself that creates the intense cravings and pressure that leads to the destructive eating habit of binging on food to satisfy pleasure or escape pain. If you don't restrict yourself in your daily diet, you lessen the cravings and conflict, which lessens your emotional need to eat.

Most nutritional experts these days recommend people eat five to six times a day (i.e. three meals and two or three snacks) every three to four hours for optimal weight management and health. Eating regularly helps keep your metabolism in calorie-burning mode. This means that your body is constantly working and is turning food into energy.

When you're eating healthy, you're eating frequently. You're just making sure that what you eat is portioned correctly. The recommendation is that half a "normal" sized plate should be taken up by vegetables and one quarter by your protein source and the other quarter by whole grains.** As a result, you feel satisfied, but never stuffed or starved.

FALSE BELIEF #2: EATING HEALTHY TASTES BAD

You have to learn that when you choose to eat healthy, this does not mean you have to eat foods like cottage cheese, grapefruit, or cabbage soup. Going on diets that promote these types of food leads people to associate eating healthy with punishment and denial. You end up believing that this is the price you have to pay if you want to lose weight. It's like you've been convicted of a crime and all you get is bread and water. This makes you devalue and dislike eating healthy.

The truth is, to lose weight you don't need to eat any food you don't like. If anything, what will help you lose weight is to eat just a normal, natural-as-possible diet that you like to eat, while watching portions and eliminating as much junk and fast food as possible. You don't have to do anything special or extreme. You don't have to eat any special "diet" foods or overhaul your entire diet.

The diets that have you eating these different types of foods that you don't normally eat, or that tell you not to eat certain foods, are just gimmicks. No elimination of one food or special combination of

---

** *In Appendix 2, you will find information about serving sizes.*

foods will help you lose weight. All you have to do is eat a balanced diet of natural food and exercise.

Does having a piece of broiled salmon with rice and vegetables and a fruit salad for dessert sound gross? You need to eat a well-balanced meal to ensure you are receiving all the nutrients you need. This means you need to eat carbs, as well as fat.

As well, there are lots of healthy desserts made with healthy ingredients that are not bad for you. For example, you could have natural Greek yogurt with some chopped up fruit, or strawberries drizzled with dark chocolate. You can have this healthy, good-tasting food every day of the week and still lose weight. As the chef Julia Child said, "the only time to eat diet food is while you're waiting for the steak to cook."

To lose weight, you can eat normal, "regular" food. All you have to do is start or go back to "traditional eating," where you have your three square meals (breakfast, lunch, and supper) made up of mostly natural food with a healthy snack and healthy dessert mixed in. That was, and still is, a healthy diet. For example, the Mediterranean diet—consisting mostly of fish, little red meat, nuts, beans, vegetables, whole grains, olive oil and fruit—has been scientifically proven to be the healthiest diet you can eat.

You can eat most of your favourite meals, just try to replace the unhealthy ingredients with healthier options. For example, use whole wheat flour instead of white flour, olive oil instead of regular oil, honey instead of sugar, butter instead of margarine.

There are also all kinds of healthy spices and sauces you can use to make your meals taste great. If you're going to eat healthy every day for the long-term, you have to like what you're eating. Experiment and have fun.

FALSE BELIEF #3: EATING HEALHY IS TIME-CONSUMING

Diet programs that provide all the frozen factory foods for you reinforce this belief that eating healthy is time-consuming. Eating healthy takes more planning and effort, but not that much more time. There is some work involved, like the cleaning and cutting up of fruit, potatoes, vegetables, and protein, stirring of pots, monitoring of cooking times, and cleaning up afterward, but not much more than that.

If you have a partner and children, divide up the work and it's even quicker. There are lots of ten to twenty-minute recipes out there, so it does not take that long to prepare and cook a healthy meal. Search the internet for ten to twenty-minute recipes and you will find hundreds.

If you can't find the time to cook and eat healthy, you have to take a look at your life and see where your time is being spent and if it can be used more wisely. The whole cooking process, including prep and clean up, can be done in under thirty minutes. For example, chopping up some vegetables and chicken, and making a stir-fry with some noodles takes no more than fifteen minutes with a less than ten minute clean up. If you were going to pick up food, by the time you drive to where you want to eat, wait in line, and drive home, it can take longer than thirty minutes.

Given the fact that Statistics Canada has said 29 per cent of Canadians over 20 spend two hours a day or more watching television, and 15 per cent at least 1.5 hours a day of their leisure time on computers—the time can be found.[47] The question is whether or not you're willing to sacrifice some entertainment time to do the task that is the most important for your well-being. It's a matter of motivation and how high it is on your priority list. Don't forget, while cooking you can still listen to music or have the television or computer on.

There are lots of ways you can make eating healthy even less time-consuming. Here is a list:

- Double up your recipes so you always have leftovers. Using leftovers for lunch saves you the time it would have taken to walk and buy fast food. As well, if you use leftovers for dinner, all you have to do is heat it up when you get home from a long day at school or work.

- Cook one-pot meals. These types of meals save on pots and dishes and are easy to cook in large amounts. For example, you could make a stew with your choice of protein, vegetables, and potatoes, or you could make a hearty soup.

- Cook one to two pots of food on your days off so you have cooked meals for the week. You can then portion out the meals so you have at least your dinners taken care of for the week and hopefully some lunches, too. This makes eating healthy a lot easier during the busy week.

- Having all the ingredients you need to cook your meals increases your chances of eating healthy. If you want to cook dinner but have to go to the grocery store first, that greatly increases the time and energy spent on preparing a healthy meal. This also makes for a good excuse to just grab some fast and easy unhealthy food.

- Buy fruits and vegetables that are easy to eat. For example, you can buy fruits like apples and bananas and vegetables like celery and cucumbers. These are good for when you're pressed for time or don't feel like cooking. It takes seconds to peel a banana and cut up some raw vegetables.

FALSE BELIEF #4:
EATING HEALTHY MEANS
YOU HAVE TO EAT PERFECT

Whenever you follow a diet program they tell you what to eat in order to lose X amount of weight in X amount of time. This means that you have to eat exactly what they say or you won't lose the weight. As previously discussed, this sets up an unrealistic expectation of having to be perfect. Having to be perfect creates the intense pressure and stress that drives you to want to eat to escape.

Having to eat perfect to lose weight also creates the intense, negative, destructive reaction when you eat more than what the diet says to. When you have a little extra food you tell yourself you have failed, so you might as well eat whatever and as much as you want. This is how you develop the destructive win-or-lose eating habit. After you're done binging, you beat yourself up and are driven to eat even more to escape.

What you have to learn is that you don't have to eat perfect to eat healthy. For example, if you eat healthy for most of the day and then eat something unhealthy, you didn't fail. One unhealthy choice does not cancel out all the previous healthy choices you made. As long as your next choice is a healthy one, it remains just one unhealthy choice.

Since we are not perfect and live in a fast-paced, hectic world, you're probably going to have to eat some processed or fast food. For example, I have a protein bar almost every day as a way of ensuring I'm getting enough protein and eating every three hours. I have some almonds and a piece of fruit with the protein bar, so that there are some natural foods mixed in.

Sometimes if I'm tired or pressed for time, I will have a

microwave dinner and a piece of fruit for dessert. If you know you have one or two days a week that are very busy, you can plan for it. This is where reading labels and finding the healthiest option you can buy becomes so important. Not all processed food is created equal, and you can find yourself eating a lot less of the bad three (saturated/trans fat, sugar, and salt) when you read the labels.***

You can also decide for yourself when you will have food that you know is not healthy, but you like. For example, maybe you decide that you're going to eat some extra food that you like on Friday or Saturday. Just knowing that you will be able to indulge a little bit one day, can help you stick to eating a healthy diet for the other six days of the week. It's not about eating perfect, it's about eating smart.

FALSE BELIEF #5: YOU ONLY EAT HEALTHY TO LOSE WEIGHT

This is the most destructive eating belief people develop. The belief that you only eat healthy to lose weight is why you always quit eating healthy once you lose weight. As mentioned earlier, eating healthy became a means to an end and becomes the price you have to pay if you want to lose weight. So when you do lose weight, you quit your diet and go back to eating for pleasure. This is why you always eventually regain your weight.

You have to learn the true value of eating healthy if you're going to make it a priority in your life. Only when you learn that eating healthy is a reward and not a punishment will you be motivated to do it for the rest of your life. If you want to treat yourself and feel pleasure, there is no better way of doing that then eating healthy.

Eating a healthy diet has way more important and positive benefits for you and your life than weight loss. Before when you tried to eat healthy, your only reason for doing so was for the benefit of your outer physical appearance. This was because you were not aware of all the inner benefits of eating healthy. Here is a list of the true benefits of eating a healthy diet:

*** *In Appendix 3 (a), you will find information about nutrition labels and how to read them and in Appendix 3 (b), you will find daily recommended nutrient amounts.*

- It improves your ability to focus your mind and think rationally and critically.

- It increases your power to control your destructive urges and emotions.

- It increases your motivation to exercise.

- It boosts your self-confidence and mood.

- It boosts your productivity and gives you energy throughout the day.

- It boosts your immune system.

- It strengthens your bones and muscles.

- It helps your organs function properly and efficiently.

- It helps you fight heart disease, diabetes, and some cancers.

- It helps increase your longevity.

- It provides structure to your day.

- It improves your sleep.

NEW HEALTHY EATING BELIEFS

These false beliefs you have developed about healthy eating has been making it harder for you to eat healthy and manage your weight. These new, true beliefs will make it easier for you to eat healthy because they are realistic and less restrictive. Instead of cravings, pressure, stress, and pain, your true rational healthy eating beliefs will create feelings of calmness, control, confidence, and pleasure.

When you learn the truth about eating healthy and change your beliefs, your reason for doing it changes. You will now want to eat healthy, because you believe it is good for you, not because you want to lose weight. Losing weight as a result of eating healthier will become a secondary benefit.

EXERCISING

Exercising, like eating healthy, is one of the pillars of living a healthy life. Unfortunately, like diet programs/products, exercise programs/products have also been advertised as producing perfect, fast, and easy weight loss and the perfect body image.

Society at large has also pushed this message that you exercise only for looks and physical power. As a result, you have also developed false and destructive beliefs about exercising. These beliefs like your false and destructive healthy eating beliefs, has been the reason you have never been able to follow an exercise routine for the long-term.

When you lost weight, you not only quit following your diet program, you also quit following your exercise program. This is because exercising was also seen as a punishment that you have to endure to lose weight, instead of being seen as the reward it is.

Just like with eating healthy, before you can learn the true benefits and pleasure of exercising, you have to first change your false, destructive beliefs about exercising. The truth will enable you to create a realistic exercise plan that will bring you true pleasure and power. Once you learn the truth about exercising, you will want to do it no matter what size you are and will never quit again. Who doesn't like to feel pleasure and power?

CHANGING YOUR FALSE BELIEFS ABOUT EXERCISING

FALSE BELIEF #1: NO PAIN, NO GAIN

The first false belief you have to break about exercising is that if you don't feel pain, you are not exercising. You've been led to believe that you have to feel pain in order to receive the benefits of exercise. A lot of people in the exercise industry push this no pain, no gain message.

You see this on reality weight loss TV shows where very overweight people who are trying to lose weight and haven't exercised in a long time are put through grueling exercise regimes by jacked-up, fitness trainers. These trainers are always yelling at the contestants to do more and telling them that they are not trying hard enough, even though you can see the pain and sweat on the peoples' faces and hear it in their grunts and groans. They're pushed to the point of collapse and exhaustion.

The Boot Camp classes that have become so popular epitomize this no pain, no gain philosophy. The name says it all. When you sign up for this type of program, you know that you are entering into a military-style of training, which is known to be extreme and intense.

Based on my experience with myself, this is not the way to motivate someone to make exercising a lifelong habit—especially somebody who is not used to exercising and is not in shape and probably doesn't like it to begin with. It's not even a safe or a healthy way to exercise. In an article about sudden, extreme exercising and the damage it can cause, it stated, "Weekend warriors and people starting a post-holiday fitness program too hard and too fast after time off are being warned that extreme exercise risks damaging the vital kidneys and muscles.[48]

You should not feel pain and exhaustion when you exercise. If you feel pain or feel like passing out, you should stop what you're doing. If not, you could hurt yourself or put your life in jeopardy. When you first start to exercise, yes, you do feel some discomfort and you struggle, but you shouldn't feel pain. Or feel like passing out.

Exercising works better when you feel energized and refreshed, both while you're doing it and when you're finished. It will leave you feeling more positive about the experience, which will motivate you to want to do it again.

When you're overweight and depressed there is already enough pain in your life. The last thing a person struggling to lose weight needs is another negative voice yelling and screaming and telling them that they are not good enough and need to do better. You don't even feel like getting out of bed some days, so it takes a lot of strength and effort to even try to exercise. This feat alone should be applauded, and you should feel proud of yourself just for trying.

Trying to exercise like an Olympian when you have barely moved your body in years is not sustainable, realistic, and most important, it's no fun. If you do not learn to like exercising, you won't be motivated to do it for the rest of your life.

The only way you will commit to exercising for the rest of your life is if you enjoy it. A long-time tennis coach discussed how he knows a child will come back to train if he can make them smile at least once during practice. This demonstrates the importance of learning how to exercise in way that will make you smile.

Exercising is more about feeling good and being healthy than being physically strong and looking good. If exercising becomes another chore in your life that you have to do but don't want to do, you will skip it or quit it when you can. This is why you have to learn that exercising is a reward. When it comes to exercising, instead of the no pain, no gain philosophy, it's the no pleasure, no forever philosophy.

FALSE BELIEF#2: YOU HAVE TO ACHIEVE A CERTAIN STANDARD OF EXCELLENCE

Following in the same vain as the no pain, no gain philosophy is the belief that you have to achieve a certain standard when you exercise. You are taught to believe that you have to lift a certain amount of weight, that you have to do a certain amount of exercises, and that you have to exercise for a certain amount of time. If you don't achieve these standards, you have failed. For example, when I was growing up if you couldn't bench press a certain weight you were considered weak.

This belief is further reinforced at school in gym class. I remember when I was going to school, every year both in public school and high school, students would be put through a national fitness test. The test involved performing a series of exercises like chin-ups, push-ups, sit-ups and sprints to see how many you could do in X amount of seconds/minutes. Then your score would be compared to some chart that would tell you if you were above average, average, or below the national fitness standard.

If you find yourself falling below the national standard of your entire country, it doesn't make you feel good about yourself or motivate you to want to exercise again. Reflect back on your own exercise and gym class experience. What standards have you tried to achieve in your exercise history?

Of course, most of the exercise ads also attach importance to numbers like how long and how many. This belief that you have to achieve these arbitrary amounts takes what is a naturally fun and enjoyable activity and turns it into something that can make you feel bad about yourself.

What you have to relearn is that there is no passing or failing when it comes to exercising. You can't be bad or fail at exercising. Exercising is simply moving your body. Just like when you were a child and ran, jumped, swam, cycled, and skipped, exercise is supposed to be fun.

There is no right amount of weight or exercises or time you have to achieve in order to be considered a powerful and fit person. The only amount you have to achieve is the amount that is right for you. Exercising is not a test you use to measure your self-worth and self-power. Don't worry about achieving some standard—just worry about doing your best and having fun.

Even Olympic athletes focus on achieving their personal best rather than winning or breaking world records. They have learned that putting pressure on yourself to win does not help your performance—it hinders it. This is because your focus is not where it needs to be.

Putting out maximum effort and trying your best is all you can control so that's where you focus all your energy. If you surpass your personal best, that shows you that you have improved and are better than you once were. What more can you ask for than that? This is victory. As long as you try your best, you can never fail.

FALSE BELIEF #3:
YOU HAVE NO TIME TO
EXERCISE/YOU HAVE TO
JOIN A GYM

These two beliefs go hand in hand in the sense that it can be time-consuming to join a gym. For example, when you join a gym you usually have to drive there, change, shower, and change again. This process can take as long or longer than your actual exercise session.

Some people like that aspect of joining a gym and use it as a place to relax and socialize. A gym can be great, but you don't have to join one to get fit. This can save you a lot of time, which seems to be everybody's issue.

The number one reason people say they don't exercise is because they don't have enough time. As mentioned earlier about the Statistics Canada findings, it seems that given the time people over 20 spend using their computers and watching television, the time can be found. If you make exercising a priority in your life, you will find and make the time.

Exercising is not as time-consuming as you have been taught and led to believe. It's a myth that you have to exercise for a certain amount of time to receive positive results. Recent research has shown that exercising for just over ten minutes a day to make up seventy-five minutes a week can produce significant health benefits.[49] Also, other research has shown that ten to fifteen minutes of exercise can boost your mood in the short-term.[50] Everyone can find ten to fifteen minutes here and there in their day to exercise. For example, you could go for a walk during your lunch break or after dinner.

As well, you can make exercise part of your daily life. For example, throughout your daily travels, when possible take the stairs instead of the elevator and walk instead of drive. When you do drive, you can also park farther away so you can walk more.

Some people carry step counters and count their daily steps. Again, an arbitrary number of ten thousand steps a day has been set as the standard you should aim for.

Whenever you are sitting down you can do mini-crunches. While you are watching television, during commercials you could do some jumping jacks or arm curls. Any type of robust cleaning or yard work can also be a form of exercise.

Every extra step you take contributes to your overall health.

The main goal of exercising should be to just try and move on a more regular and consistent basis. Think about your life and figure out where you can make exercising a part of your daily routine.

FALSE BELIEF #4: LIFTING WEIGHTS WILL MAKE YOU BULKY

A lot of people have the false belief that lifting weights makes you bulky. For people who are trying to lose weight, the last thing they want is to become even bigger.

As soon as people think about lifting weights, they think about the body builders on the cover of those weight lifting magazines. That is not how building and strengthening your muscles naturally works. For most people, the only way you get that big is by taking steroids. The truth is, people who are naturally bigger will grow big muscles and people who are smaller will grow muscles suited for their body frame.

Also, you can lift weights in a manner that emphasizes definition over growth. For example, you lift lighter weights and do more reps (8-12) for sculpting and you lift heavier weights and do fewer reps (4-6) for greater size.

What working out with weights does do is help to change the composition of your body. Strength training changes fat into muscle and gives your body shape and tone. This is why you cannot pay too much attention to what the scale says when you're lifting weights regularly.

A pound of muscle and a pound of fat weigh the same, but muscles are denser and so take up less space. So even though you did not lose weight, you are smaller. This is why it's better to measure yourself than to weigh yourself. It's a truer measurement of physical change. Since muscles take up less space than fat, you could say that gaining muscles will actually make you smaller, not bulkier.

In addition, when you lift weights, you break down your muscles and then your muscles have to repair themselves. While your muscles are repairing and rebuilding themselves, your body continues to work, which keeps you in calorie-burning mode. This helps you burn extra weight. All you have to do is set the process in motion by adding strength training to your exercise routine.

FALSE BELIEF #5:
YOU ONLY EXERCISE TO
LOSE WEIGHT

As a result of listening to society and exercise ads, you believe the only reason you exercise is to lose weight. Whenever you exercise all your focus is on losing weight and trying to achieve the perfect body image. You exercise as hard as you can and as long as you can, so you can lose as much weight as fast as possible. Your results are measured by how you look in the mirror and by how much you weigh on the scale.

What you need to learn is that exercising is as good for your inner mind and body as it is for your physical appearance. For example, exercising helps improve the functioning of your brain. It increases the blood/oxygen flow to your brain, which increases the powers of your higher thinking faculties. This enables you to focus and think more rationally and make better decisions and choices.

Exercising also helps to make you feel even better about who you are. When you make the healthy choice to exercise, it boosts your self-confidence. By achieving your daily goals and making choices you rationally know is good for your health and well-being makes you feel powerful and in control of yourself and life. This increases your positive thinking. In an article by Psychology Today.com it stated, "Exercise elevates mood by psychological means as well as physiological ones. It changes people's perception of themselves, providing a sense of personal mastery. It also reduces negative thinking."[51]

As well, exercising makes you feel pleasure. When you exercise, pleasure chemicals known as endorphins are released that make you feel good. If you're stressed or depressed, exercising will boost your mood and energy. Kristen Vickers-Douglas, Ph.D., a psychologist at Mayo Clinic, Rochester, Minn says, "it's not a magic bullet, but increasing physical activity is a positive and active strategy to help manage depression and anxiety."[52]

By exercising, you also take your mind off your problems and let your body do the work. It gives your mind a chance to shut off and be quiet. Most of the time you're in your head, worrying about this and reacting to that. It feels good to get out of your head for a while and focus on something else. In an article by Mayoclinic.com, it included distraction as one of the numerous psychological and emotional benefits of exercising if you have depression or anxiety, and said that, "when you have depression or anxiety, it's easy to dwell on how badly you feel. But dwelling interferes with your ability to problem solve and cope in a healthy way. Dwelling also can make depression more severe and longer lasting. Exercise can provide a good distraction. It shifts the focus away from the unpleasant thoughts to something more pleasant, such as your surroundings or the music you enjoy listening to while you exercise."[53]

There can be a lot of daily stress, upset, and frustration in life. Exercising allows you to de-stress and burn off all that built-up negative energy. It helps you to purify your mind and body. As Nicki Anderson, a personal trainer stated, "In short the biggest reason to exercise is sanity."[54]

Even if you are already feeling good and doing good, after exercising you will feel even better and will perform even better in every aspect of your life. For example, you will have more energy and enthusiasm at work and at play. You have to learn for yourself that nothing makes you feel more pleasure and more power than when you make the choice to exercise. When you learn for yourself that exercising makes you feel good mentally, psychologically, emotionally, spiritually, and physically, you will be more motivated to do it.

Yes, exercising helps you burn some calories and lose some weight, but there are so many more important reasons why you should exercise. Here is a list of some more reasons why you should make the choice to exercise and not one of them has anything to do with losing weight and how you look:

- It boosts your immune system and helps you fight diseases like diabetes and some cancers.

- It increases your longevity.

- It adds structure to your day.

- It helps prevent boredom and impulsive behaviour.

- It motivates you to eat healthy.

- It helps you sleep better.

- It helps you drink more water.

- It gives you a way of honouring yourself and your Creator by showing gratitude for what you have (e.g., your body is your temple).

- It allows you to have the best day possible.

NEW EXERCISE BELIEFS

When you learn the truth about exercising and change your beliefs, your reason for exercising will also change. Just like with eating healthy, instead of exercising to lose weight, you will now exercise to feel good holistically. As well, your new, true rational exercise beliefs will make it easier for you to say yes to exercising and harder for you to say no.

Now that you have changed your false and destructive beliefs about why and how to eat healthy and exercise, it's time to learn what's the best approach to use that will help you create a healthy living plan you can follow for the long-term.

CHANGING YOUR APPROACH TO LIVING HEALTHY

THE SLOW, STEADY, STEP-BY-STEP, TRY-YOUR-BEST APPROACH

Since you have learned that the perfect, fast, and easy diet and exercise approach is not the path to weight loss success, you will be more open to trying a new approach. The path to success is the exact opposite of the approach you were using. Instead of the perfect, fast, and easy approach, it's time to try the slow, steady, step-by-step, try-your-best approach.

When you use this type of approach, your attention will be focused on your inner self and feeling pleasure and power, not on your outer self and how much weight you have to lose in X amount of time. All you have to do is try and make one or two healthy changes to how you eat and how you move and focus your attention on how good it makes you feel holistically. When you're comfortable and are in the habit of performing the new changes consistently, then you make more. It's this rational and realistic approach that will help you live a healthier lifestyle, and as a result will help you lose and manage your weight.

THE PHILOSOPHY OF SLOW

When you first try to make changes to your behaviour, the best approach, is the slow one. Since you no longer have to achieve the perfect body to love and accept yourself, there is no rush or deadline. There's no longer a need or value-priority to lose X amount of weight, in X amount of time. As a result, you can take your foot off the pedal and just breathe, relax, and take your time. This allows you to focus your mind on learning, growing, and enjoying the process of making positive changes to your behaviour and life.

When you're taking it slow all your focus is on slowing down the thoughts in your mind, relaxing your body, and remaining calm. Your focus and attention is on the moment and the behaviour you are performing. While you're performing your behaviour, you move slow, you think slow, and you breath slow. For example, when you lift weights, you lift in a slow and controlled way. You're not thinking about how much weight or how many or the next movements you have to do. Instead, you're focused on your form and how good it feels to move your body in the moment. This is the opposite of rushing through an exercise and thinking about the next five exercises you have to do in order to lose weight fast. This creates unnecessary anxiety and stress, which makes you not enjoy what you're doing.

Even if you're going for a run on a treadmill, you do it in a slow and relaxed way. For example, you can set the speed at a rate that allows you to control your movements and your breathing. If you're too out of breath to do this, you know you're going too fast and too hard. If you want, you could just do Tai chi which is an exercise practice based on slow movement and slow breathing.

In regards to following your healthy eating plan, you focus on one meal and movement at a time. The prep, cooking, and cleaning is all done in a slow, controlled, conscious manner. You only think about your next meal, when you're scheduled time to eat arrives, versus, thinking about having to eat perfect for the whole day. For example, when prepping your food, instead of focusing on how much work there is and how much more cooking you have to do, focus on enjoying the moment. Slow your mind and body down and pay attention to how the knife feels in your hand, the motion of chopping, the sound of the food, and how good it feels to just be alive and doing in the moment.

By moving consciously and slowly, and focusing your mind on what you're doing in the moment, you learn that this helps reduce stress and helps you feel calm and even joy. When you're calm and happy, that means you're enjoying what you're doing. You learn that it feels good to quiet your mind and perform a task in a slow and calm manner.

Since you're moving slow and are cool, calm, and collected, your actions are methodical and precise. As a result, you will make fewer mistakes. The opposite is true for when you're rushing. For example, if you're cooking dinner in a rush, the chances increase that you will cut yourself or break or drop something. Just like if you're rushing while you exercise, you increase your chances of injuring yourself.

Unless it's truly a life-or-death situation, there is no need to rush. It's a myth that rushing saves time or produces greater results. When you're rushing, your mind is frazzled which leads to mistakes and having to go over things again. You just end up going around in circles. As the saying goes, "slow and steady wins the race." This is especially true for life, which is not a race, but a marathon. If you go too fast and too hard, you will burn out and won't be able to reach the finish line. Why create unnecessary anxiety and stress in your life? Take it easy on yourself and take it slow. You will be happier and more productive.

PROCESS VERSUS RESULTS

Contrary to what you have been taught by the diet industry, changing your behaviour is not easy and does not happen overnight. Successful behaviour change takes hard work, patience, perseverance, practice, persistence, and passion. Mistakes will be made repeatedly and frustration will be felt. It's this knowledge and mindset that will help you achieve your goals and dreams.

As you have learned, you developed a lot of destructive emotional eating habits that make it hard for you to eat healthy and lose weight. You have to learn about each one of these habits and why you do them before you can break them. Only then will you have a chance of following your healthy eating plan consistently.

Also, you live in an obesogenic environment so there is temptation everywhere. In one study of a suburb in Canada, ninety-two fast food outlets were found within a three kilometre radius.[55]

Overcoming all your temptations and destructive emotional eating behaviours is a process of failing, learning, and trying again. Learning to break old, unhealthy habits and learning to adopt new, healthy habits takes time. I like the advice given by dietitian Andrea Holwegner: "Trying something new and getting into a healthy eating groove takes time and patience. Repetition is needed to develop any new habit, so cut yourself some slack and remember that anything new feels awkward until you get into the habit. The first time you try adding a piece of fruit to your usual breakfast of toast and peanut butter won't feel just right. How could it when you have never done it before? But after you have repeated this new awkward habit over time, it becomes second nature. Acknowledge that change, no matter how small, is hard."[56]

Losing weight is not about willing yourself to achieve some result it's about learning how to overcome your destructive habits and live a healthy life. When you fail to eat as healthy as you wanted or don't exercise, the point is to learn why you made those choices so you can learn about yourself and what to do the next time so you don't make the same mistake again. Reacting emotionally and beating yourself up and putting more pressure on yourself after you fail doesn't help. It's not productive; instead, it's counterproductive. Again, it just creates more intense, toxic, negative emotions which triggers you to want to binge and escape.

Learning why you fail is a big part of your future success. As the wise say, "In order to win, you have to lose." It's as important as learning what works. For diet programs/products to make claims of weight loss without teaching people how to cope with their unhealthy eating habits is irresponsible, negligible, and downright dangerous.

As long as you continue to keep on learning and trying your best to eat healthy and exercise, you can never lose or feel too bad about yourself. Only you can look yourself in the mirror and know if you are trying your best. You have to believe that as long as you are, you will improve. You have to trust the process, no matter what the scale says.

BABY STEPS

The ideal goal of any healthy living plan is to eat an all-natural diet and to exercise daily. Although this is where you might want to end up, this is not where you start. It's mostly unrealistic to think you can go from an unhealthy lifestyle to a healthy lifestyle overnight (due to the reasons discussed above). You have to crawl before you can walk.

Attempting to live a one hundred percent healthy life and lose lots of weight is something you have to slowly work up to. Overhauling your entire life (after months/years of living unhealthy) all at once and expecting immediate transformation is overwhelming, which is what makes it difficult. This is the opposite of how you need to think and feel in order to be successful.

As discussed, trying to implement these unrealistic, extreme changes to your behaviour in order to achieve fast and easy weight loss creates cravings, pressure, stress, and pain, all which trigger you to want to binge. The best thing you can do to prevent this from happening is to incrementally introduce practical, realistic changes into your daily life.

To make positive and significant changes to your overall health and well-being, there is no need to overhaul your entire lifestyle and follow a rigid and restrictive plan perfectly. By trying to achieve only one or two changes to how you eat and move, you can decrease the stress and increase the success. This is because you have to only focus on making a small amount of changes and don't have to be perfect all at once. All your attention can be focused on making some changes, instead of worrying about having to change everything.

Having small, manageable goals you can achieve increases your belief you can be successful. When you're successful at making one change, it increases your motivation to make another change. Every change you make boosts your self-confidence, cuts calories, and contributes to living a healthier lifestyle.

In the previous mentioned Mayoclinic.com article, one of the tips it gave to help you exercise when you have depression or anxiety is to set reasonable goals. It stated, "Your mission doesn't have to be walking for an hour five days a week. Think about what you may be able to do in reality. Twenty minutes? Ten minutes? Start there and build up. Custom-tailor your plan to your own needs and abilities rather than trying to meet idealistic guidelines that could just add to your pressure."[57]

Even the most decorated Olympic gold medalist swimmer Michael Phelps discussed in an interview that after taking six months off, it took him a year and a half to get back to the level he was. He had to start off slow and build himself back up step-by-step.

If you haven't exercised for a long time, it's unrealistic to think you will be able to exercise every day of the week. Instead, you could try to exercise two days a week. You could do one cardio session one day and one strength training session on another day. If you are having trouble keeping up with this amount, why stress yourself out thinking about having to exercise for seven days? Once you prove to yourself that you can do two days, you can then add another day and so on.

When it comes to eating healthy, instead of trying to follow a new seven-day diet plan that contains a bunch of foods you have never cooked or eaten before, try a three-day plan and try to cook one healthy meal a day that you like and know how to make. For example, if you eat a lot of processed and fast food, start by trying to have one meal a day that is natural, like having a piece of fish with a baked potato, vegetables, and a piece of fruit for dessert. By substituting one bad meal with one good meal a day, you can make a big difference to your overall health.****

Along with substituting one unhealthy meal with a healthy meal, you could also try to cut your junk food/drink intake by half, instead of trying to eliminate it all at once. This is a more practical, doable, and most importantly, a less stressful approach.

These are great first steps to living a more healthy life. You can continue to make changes until you are eating an almost all-natural healthy diet and are exercising daily.

SMALL CHANGE IS BIG CHANGE

By following and listening to the majority of diet and exercise programs, people are led to believe that they can and should lose a lot of weight fast. The truth is, it's not safe or healthy to lose a lot of weight fast, and it's definitely not sustainable. You can only do extreme for so long before you return to your normal way of eating and living.

The consensus among the medical profession seems to be that losing any more than a pound or two a week is unhealthy. As Dr. Lance Levy stated in his book, *Conquering Obesity*, "Clients who are losing more than 2.2 pounds (1 kg) a week are going too quickly. Very drastic diets may produce more rapid changes in body-water balance (dehydration), but the rate will ultimately slow down (plateau) and you will lose much-needed muscle tissue as well as water and excess body fat. Clients say that they are doing these diets for a couple of weeks only, perhaps to get ready for a party, and that therefore they can suffer no real harm. I don't agree. During weight loss it is important to allow changes in body composition to occur fairly slowly and try to preserve muscle mass by combining a well-balanced diet with exercise."[58]

Dr. Lance Levy also stated that for someone who has been obese for a long time, a five to ten percent change in their body mass can make not only a significant difference to how they feel and move but also lessen the risk of cardiovascular disease and getting diabetes.[59] This seems to add to the evidence that small changes can have big results, and you don't need to resort to drastic measures to lose weight.

**** *In Appendix 4, is an example of a starter meal plan and starter exercise program.*

CONSISTENCY, CONSISTENCY, CONSISTENCY

What is most important when you're trying to make new lifestyle changes is how consistently you do it. As you know, you can eat healthy and exercise for three months and lose lots of weight but after you quit, all the positive results quickly disappear.

The number of exercise programs I did for a few months and quit equals up to multiple years, but because it was start-and-stop, I didn't see any long lasting results.

I've heard it said and have experienced it for myself that it's around a 3:1 ratio when it comes to how long it takes for results to disappear. This means if you exercise for three months, it will take a month for the benefits to ware off.

To avoid this start-stop outcome, your short-term goal should be to make small changes to your lifestyle that you can follow on a daily basis and your long-term goal should be to try to maintain your changes for a year. This is so you can get yourself into the routine of eating healthy and exercising. For instance, if you were able to follow the one healthy meal a day (plus lessening your junk food/drink intake) and the one cardio and one strength-training a week plan for a year (plus adding extra movements into your daily life), you would definitely lose weight, but more importantly you would have established a long-term habit of making healthy choices.

As well, after living a healthier lifestyle for a year, you would have proved to yourself that you can trust yourself to keep a commitment and can achieve your short and long-term goals. This will increase your belief in yourself and your abilities.

Also, you would have given yourself the time to learn for yourself how pleasurable eating healthy, exercising, and following a routine feels. Which, will motivate you to make more healthy changes to your life.

FOLLOWING YOUR NEW, TRUE, RATIONAL BELIEF SYSTEM

Once you have changed your old approach and old beliefs, and have adopted a new approach, a new belief system, and a new healthy living plan, the next thing to figure out is how you're going to follow what you changed. To be able to follow your new changes on a consistent basis, you're going to have to break all the destructive emotional eating habits you have developed. To accomplish this, you have to learn for yourself that by following your new, true, rational beliefs, rational approach, and rational healthy living plan, you have the power to cope with your own emotions and can bring yourself greater relief from pain and greater pleasure than binging on food can. This is how you will learn that there is nothing more valuable and important than your mind and the rational truth.

You can rationally believe that your beliefs, approach, and plan are true, but in order to live by them, you're going to have to prove to yourself that they are valuable as well. To value something, you have to like it or at least appreciate it.

Learning what truly brings you success and pleasure and what truly brings you failure and pain, involves rationally and critically re-evaluating your values and behaviour. Changing your false, destructive beliefs step one in changing your feelings and behaviour. The second step is changing your false, destructive values.

PART THREE:
LIFESTYLE RECONSTRUCTION

(The putting together of a healthy life)

CHAPTER 14 :

CHANGING YOUR VALUE SYSTEM

VALUES AND BEHAVIOUR

It's great to have beliefs, but without the action, it's just blah, blah, blah. The question always comes down to, "Yes, you can talk the talk, but can you walk the walk?" As the saying goes, "Talk is cheap and that actions speak louder than words." The difficulty of doing what you say is expressed in author Mark Twain's statement, "Action speaks louder than words but not nearly as often."

You can say to yourself that you believe in your rational, true beliefs, approach, and healthy living plan, but what are you going to do when you fail and are confronted by your feelings of depression and are triggered to want to quit and binge on food to escape, or are in the face of temptation and feel your intense cravings? Will you be able to follow what you rationally believe, or will you give in to your strong desire to binge on food? This is the heart of the matter and what makes following your rational beliefs a challenge. At some point, you're going to have to prove to yourself that you believe in your beliefs and can follow them no matter how strong and intense your urge to binge on food to feel pleasure or escape pain is.

Although you have gone through the process of learning what is true, you will still be confronted and challenged by all the emotional eating habits you developed. As discussed in part one, you became dependent on food to both satisfy your cravings and to escape the negative emotions and pain you experienced due to following and failing at the perfect, fast, and easy diet approach. As a result, you learned to value binging on food to satisfy pleasure and to escape pain. This is how binging on food became the way you cope with your emotions.

You have to remember that some of your destructive eating habits go back to birth and childhood. For example, we are born to like fatty, salty, and sugary foods and when younger, we are rewarded with fatty, salty, and sugary foods if we behave good and it's withheld if we behave badly.

As well, since most people start dieting before they are teens, and depending on how old you are these destructive emotional eating habits could be twenty years old. They are strong and ingrained, and they are going nowhere. They must be understood fully if you're going to be able to follow what you rationally believe.

Also, as you learned, due to the restrictions and unrealistic expectations of the perfect, fast, and easy diet approach, you learned to devalue and hate eating healthy. This is why you quit doing it once you successfully lose weight.

To change your behaviour for the long-term, you're going to have to change your values (what you love and what you hate). You love and value what brings you pleasure and hate and devalue what brings you pain. You will only do a behaviour you hate, if you learn to love it and you will only stop doing a behaviour you love, if you learn to hate it.

INSIGHT

In order to be able to follow your rational beliefs on a consistent basis, you're going to have to fight and break all of your emotional eating habits. To accomplish this feat, you're going to have to scrutinize each bad habit and become intimately aware of the automatic, emotional reactions and urges that trigger them.

Most times, you just react to your impulse to binge on food to escape pain or feel pleasure without knowing what is causing it. By trying to understand internally what causes you to feel and act destructively is how you will gain insight into yourself/mind and your behaviour. This insight will help you become aware of the destructive reactions and urges that are driving you to feel and act destructively. Once you have this self-knowledge, you will have the power to change how you feel and behave.

Additionally, you have to prove to yourself that the short-term pleasure or pain-relief that your emotional eating habits might bring you, is not worth the long-term pain you experience. To learn this truth, every time you give in to one of your emotional eating habits you have to evaluate your experience. You do this by asking yourself if the short-term pleasure or pain relief you felt was worth the long-term pain you feel. When you learn its true value, you will not value it as much and, therefore, will not want to do it as much.

What will further help you break your destructive emotional

eating habits and make you value following your new beliefs, approach, and plan is learning for yourself that by doing so, you have the power to control and change your destructive emotional reactions and urges, and can make yourself feel greater pleasure and greater pain relief than binging on food. This is how you learn that following your rational beliefs, rational approach, and rational healthy living plan is a better way of coping with your destructive feelings than binging on food.

To learn these truths about what is good for you and what is bad for you, your focus needs to be on your inner mind and body. By paying attention to your inner mind and body is how you will learn for yourself that it's the false and destructive beliefs, thoughts, and evaluations in your mind that are creating the destructive feelings that drive you to act destructively. It's also how you learn for yourself that by changing the false with the rational truth you can make yourself feel better and behave better.

As well, you have to be focused on your inner mind and body to learn that following your emotional eating habits to seek pleasure or escape negative emotions and pain only brings you long-term pain, and that eating healthy and exercising only brings you long-term pleasure, power, and relief. This is where you look to learn the true consequences of your behaviour, not by looking at the numbers on a scale.

MINDFULNESS

To assist you in learning about the destructive thoughts, beliefs, and evaluations that trigger your destructive emotional eating habits and how following the rational truth can change how you feel and behave for the better, you have to practice mindfulness. The technique of mindfulness was first practiced in the cultures of South and Southeast Asia over 2, 500 years ago.[60]

Mindfulness helps one gain honest insight into what thoughts, beliefs, evaluations, and behaviours bring you pleasure and success and what thoughts, beliefs, evaluations, and behaviours bring you pain and failure. By learning this knowledge you are able to discover how to think and act in order to feel good.

Buddhist monk H. Gunaratana Mahathera in his book about the Vipassana meditation practice which uses the technique of mindfulness, explained it like this: "We are going to teach you to watch the functioning of your own mind in a calm and detached manner so you can gain insight into your own behaviour. The goal is awareness, an awareness so intense, concentrated and finely tuned that you will be able to pierce the inner workings of reality itself."[61]

To be mindful, you have to observe yourself like an impartial, neutral, rational scientist. This means that you keep your personal biases and feelings out of it and let the empirical evidence speak for itself. You study yourself like you would any other subject studied in school. It's all about learning the facts. Instead of being a school examination, this is a self-examination.

To learn the truth about why you feel and act the way you do, you have to rationally and critically observe what is happening inside your body and mind. To do this, you have to be focused on and aware of your inner self. For example, by being mindful you will become aware that after failing you feel toxic emotions and feel like binging to escape. To find out why you feel the way you do, you check your mind to find out what you were just saying to yourself. What you will find is that you were making negative statements and calling yourself negative names. By repeatedly being mindful, you will start to see that your negative reaction to failing is causing you pain and self-destruction and needs to be changed.

If you find yourself becoming caught up in your emotions or are judging yourself harshly for your reaction, stop yourself and go back to being the silent observer and rational learner. All you are interested in and focused on is paying attention to what is going on inside of your body and mind, so you can learn what is causing you to feel and act the way you do. You're not doing it to condemn yourself for the way you think, feel, and act.

REFLECTIVE MINDFULNESS

When you first study yourself to learn why you feel and act the way you do, you usually do become caught up in your reactions and urges, and have to be mindful after the fact. Your emotional reactions and urges are automatic and strong, and so is your habit to eat to escape or feel pleasure. As a result, many times you find yourself asking, "Why did I just eat?" This is when you have to practice reflective mindfulness and do a post-performance, play-by-play analysis.

You have to ask yourself questions like, "What was the situation?," "What was I feeling in my body prior to acting?," and "What was going on inside my mind?"/ "What was I thinking?" By doing this, you can learn why you behaved the way you did, and what situations, thoughts, and feelings you have to look out for and correct. For example, you might discover that you ate because you saw a food ad on television and you automatically told yourself, "I want some, it would be good," and felt your cravings in your body and automatically binged. So the next time you're watching television and see a food ad, you know to be mindful and to watch for physical cues (licking lips) and mental cues (fantasizing about food) that you are being triggered by your cravings. This will help you to stop and change your destructive emotional reaction before you automatically satisfy your urge to eat.

By practicing reflective mindfulness you can also do value-comparisons to evaluate your value-choices. For example, when you choose to make the value-choice to follow your rational beliefs, rational approach, and rational healthy living plan, you can pay attention to your mind and body to learn how much pleasure and pain relief you feel compared to the painful experience you have when you choose to follow your feelings and eat unhealthy. This is how you can learn that the short-term pain of denying yourself immediate pleasure or pain relief, is worth it for the long-term pleasure, power, and relief you feel. On the other hand, you learn that binging on food to experience short-term pleasure or short-term relief is not worth the inner long-term psychological, physical, and mental pain you feel. This is the only way you can learn that not all pain is bad and not all pleasure is good. It's an important lesson to learn since seeking pleasure and avoiding pain is a natural instinct.

SELF-AWARENESS

When you rationally know the true value of things for yourself, you now have the power to fight what you automatically love and hate and can instead make the conscious, rational value-choices you know through experience lead to long-term pleasure and power. When you start making daily, conscious, rational value-choices you regain control over your self and your weight. Your self and weight start to balance out. There is less reacting to your strong emotions and urges, and more inner stability as you remain focused on your mind and the rational truth. As a result, you feel more calm and rational and feel less emotional and irrational.

You have to go through this process of rationally and critically observing, evaluating, and comparing your reactions and value-choices to become aware of what is truly bringing you pleasure and success and what is truly bringing you pain and failure. This is how you can resolve your inner value-conflicts and reprioritize your values. It's also how you can go from having to do the right thing, to wanting to do it.

In the next chapter, you will learn a technique that will help you control and change your body once you become aware that you have been emotionally triggered. As well, you will learn a technique to help you control, challenge, and change your mind to the rational truth, so you can change how you feel and act. The goal is to help you learn how to control and change your mind and body once you become aware you have been emotionally triggered. This is so you will be able to stop yourself from reacting emotionally and destructively, and instead, refocus on the rational truth and act thoughtfully and wisely. This is what can help you cope with your destructive emotional reactions and urges and break all of your destructive emotional eating habits.

CHAPTER 15:

CHANGING YOUR DEPRESSION EATING HABIT

Let's begin the process of changing your destructive emotional eating habits by examining how you react to being overweight again. When you're in the rock bottom stage, the first destructive emotional eating habit you have to learn to cope with is eating to escape feelings of depression.

As discussed, you hit rock bottom because you were unable to stop yourself from gaining all the weight you originally lost. Your mind is consumed with negative self-evaluations, and your body is consumed by feelings of depression and the pain of overeating. Every time you think about, feel, or see the weight you gained, you feel worthless, powerless, hopeless, and as a result, depressed. All you feel like doing is binging and escaping.

COGNITIVE BEHAVIOURAL THERAPY

Before you learned the truth about the diet approach and yourself, you would just accept your rock bottom self-evaluations as being true and would react to your negative feelings by binging on food to escape. You now have the power of the rational truth on your side and can challenge and change your false self-evaluations.

By challenging your irrational evaluations with the rational truth, you can make yourself feel better about yourself, which will motivate you to continue to fight to stick to your healthy living plan. This is how you will begin to learn the truth that by controlling your mind, you have the power to control how you feel and act.

To help you challenge and change the false, destructive thoughts, beliefs, and evaluations that are causing you to feel and eat destructively, you can use a therapeutic technique called cognitive behavioural therapy (CBT), also known as self-talk therapy. CBT is commonly used by psychologists, therapists, and counsellors who work with people suffering from depression. They use CBT to help people gain insight into the fact that it's how they are talking to themselves in their head that is making them feel and act the way they do. The hope is that once people become aware of this, they can learn to challenge and change their negative self-talk to the truth, and thus change the depressive feelings that trigger their destructive behaviour. Besides treating depression, cognitive therapy has also been shown to be effective in treating other emotional disorders, addiction issues, eating disorders, and relationship problems.[62]

Your urge to escape your feelings of depression are so strong and intense that you often give in to them without questioning them. This is why you binge every day for weeks, sometimes months. You end up eating because you're depressed and you're depressed because you eat. These feelings take over your entire being. You feel you have no other choice but to binge to escape your reality and how you feel. If you want to change your destructive emotional reaction to being overweight and depressed you're going to have to start to ask yourself, "Why do I feel the way I do?"

Feelings do not just appear out of thin air and are not evidence that confirm your thinking. For example, a lot of people believe they must be worthless or else they wouldn't feel worthless. The truth is, it's the exact opposite—feelings are the result of your thoughts and evaluations. If you feel worthless, it's because you evaluated yourself as such. As has been stated many times, how you think is how you feel. To feel positive and act positive, you have to use CBT to challenge and change your false, negative, irrational self-talk into true, positive, rational self-talk.

When you use CBT, you're not just observing your self-talk, you're questioning its validity. Unless it's a truly life-or-death situation that demands immediate action, all feelings and impulses have to be rationally and critically challenged before acting on them. It's the only way to ensure your feelings are justified and that your actions will bring you pleasure and success. You have to ask yourself questions like, Why am I feeling this way? Will my behaviour bring me pleasure or pain? and Is my thinking true or false? If you find that your self-talk is false, you can then change your self-talk to the rational truth and change how you feel and act. This is what it means to be a thoughtful person, rather than an impulsive, emotional person.

DEEP BREATHING EXERCISES

One way you can slow down the automatic, strong, emotional reactions and urges you feel so you can think rationally and critically before acting, is to do some deep breathing exercises. Since your evaluations and impulses happen fast, they are usually first felt in your body in the form of physiological changes. For example, your heart beats faster and your breathing quickens. It's usually in the body that you first become aware that you have been emotionally triggered.

Whenever you become aware that your emotions are taking over your body and behaviour, close your eyes and focus your attention on your breathing. Take a deep breath in through your nose or mouth until your lungs are full and then take a long, slow, deep breathe out through your nose or mouth, and repeat. You continue to do this until your body is relaxed, your mind is quiet, and your emotions are calm, centred, and balanced.

By engaging in deep breathing, it helps to stop/slow down the automatic, strong, physiological reaction that happens in your body when you're triggered emotionally. When you try to slow down your breathing, your focus changes from reacting to how you feel to controlling how you breathe. This temporarily takes your focus off your emotional reaction and your urge to eat to escape.

Focusing on your breathing grounds you back into the present moment. It brings you back into a state of awareness and mind/body control. This is what gives you the chance to think rationally. As Buddhist and famous spiritual author Thich Nhat Hanh wrote, "as you breathe in, you can connect with your body. Bring your mind home to your body and remember that you have a body. Very often we're carried far away by our thinking; we're caught by sorrow and regret concerning the past, by fear and anxiety concerning the future, or by our emotions or projects in the present. Our mind is not with our body."[63]

CHALLENGING YOUR MIND

Whenever you are being mindful and notice you feel depressed (deep anguish, deep sighs, sobs, head down, low mood, no energy, no motivation) or hear yourself say, "I'm depressed" and are triggered to eat to escape, do some deep breathing. Once calm and in control, turn your attention to your mind and check to see what you were saying to yourself. When you do, you will discover you were repeating your rock bottom self-evaluations to yourself and saying statements like:

- I'm not acceptable.

- I'm not worthy.

- I'm a failure.

- I'm cursed.

To make yourself feel better so you don't have to binge on food to escape your feelings of depression, remind yourself of your true, rational beliefs. Remind yourself that:

- You accept and love yourself unconditionally.

- You are so much more than your body image and that you are worthy as is. Tell yourself the reasons why.

- You are powerful and can control how you feel and act. Tell yourself the reasons why.

- You are blessed. Count them one by one.

Be mindful and focus on how repeatedly telling yourself the rational truth makes you feel better and motivates you to fight your urge to eat to escape. When you feel acceptable, worthy, powerful, hopeful, and happy, you have the energy and motivation to make positive value-choices—like following your healthy living plan. Remember, saying self-affirmations has the power to make you feel good.

CHANGING YOUR MIND

By controlling your breathing and challenging your rock bottom self-evaluations with the truth, you stop yourself from automatically satisfying your urge to binge on food to escape. You give yourself an opportunity to speak some sense into yourself before acting destructively. Once your mind is focused on the rational truth, you feel positive and now want to make the positive value-choices that will help you continue to feel good. All you need to give yourself is that split second for your rational thinking to regain control over how you feel and act.

Every time you challenge and change your automatic, false,

rock bottom self-evaluations that are causing you to feel the depressive feelings that trigger you to want to binge to escape with your new, true, rational beliefs and end up feeling better and eating better, the stronger this behaviour becomes. You have to continue to do this until following your rational self-beliefs when you feel depressed and feel like binging becomes a habit. By then you would have proven to yourself that your rational self-beliefs are not only true, but valuable.

VALUE-CHOICE COMPARISON

Be mindful and compare this experience to when you make the value-choice to react to your feelings of depression by binging on food to escape. Pay attention to how you feel physically, mentally, and psychologically. What you will find is that after you're done binging on food, your rock bottom self-evaluations are stronger and you feel even more depressed and feel even more food hangover pain. Since your feelings of depression and pain are stronger (because you failed and overate), it's now harder for you to focus your mind on following the rational truth. This is because your mind is filled with the negative and destructive evaluations that create the destructive feelings triggering your urge to binge to escape.

The worse you feel, the stronger your urge to binge and escape is, and the lower your energy and motivation to follow your healthy living plan is. You end up not feeling like it. All you do feel like doing is eating and escaping.

Now, when you binge on food to medicate yourself from your intense feelings of depression you are able to numb yourself from the pain for a short while. So, you have to ask yourself if the increased feelings of depression and pain you feel later is worth it. If you are rationally and honestly evaluating your experience, the answer would be no.

Going through this process of comparing the consequences of your value-choices is how you learn that making the value-choice to follow your true, rational self-beliefs is a better way of coping with your feelings of depression than making the value-choice to binge on food to escape. This is how you can break your dysfunctional and destructive emotional eating habit of binging on food when you feel depressed. It's also how you start to learn to value controlling your mind and body to make yourself feel and do better.

CHANGING YOUR HABIT OF QUITTING WHEN YOU FAIL

The other rock bottom reaction you need to challenge and change is what you tell yourself when you first try to eat healthy and exercise again and fail. How you have reacted in the past has made your depression worse and triggered you to quit trying and instead binge on food for a long duration.

Since you're not perfect, combined with the fact that your feelings of depression and pain are strong, and you're in the habit of eating to escape, there will be times when you fail to follow your true beliefs and healthy living plan. You will instead follow your negative self-talk and surrender to your urge to escape your negative and painful feelings.

CHALLENGING AND CHANGING YOUR MIND

Whenever you overeat to escape feelings of depression, be mindful and if you notice you're feeling more depressed and wanting to quit and binge, do some deep breathing. Then reflect on what you were saying to yourself. When you do, you will discover that you were singing the "woe is me" blues and telling yourself things like:

- What's the point of trying?

- I can't, I won't, I'll never lose weight.

- I'm no good.

- I'm a failure.

- I'm cursed.

- I suck and my life sucks.

After this type of negative reaction to failing, you now feel even more worthless, helpless, and hopeless, which increases your feelings of depression and desire to quit trying. As discussed in part one, when you lose your internal locus of control and believe you have no power to change yourself and life for the better, you lose the motivation to try. This is why you wave the white flag, surrender, and go on a "bender."

To change your rock bottom reaction to failing, you have to once again engage in some self-talk therapy. You learn for yourself that if you don't want to give up and quit, you have to fight your emotional reactions with the rational truth. Remind yourself that:

- You forgive yourself for failing because it's not your fault you developed these destructive emotional eating habits.

- You accept and love yourself as is.

- You believe you can and will succeed.

- You are blessed.

- Quitting only makes things worse and is how you gain lots of weight.

- You are not perfect and that failing and learning from your mistakes is part of the process of trying to change your behaviour.

Again, be mindful and pay attention to how reminding yourself of your true, rational beliefs makes you feel worthy, powerful, and hopeful and gives you the strength and motivation to pick yourself back up faster and try again. You learn for yourself that if you don't want to give up and quit, you have to fight your emotional reactions with the rational truth.

VALUE-COMPARISON

Now, when you make the value-choice to quit and eat unhealthy for an extended period of time after failing, be mindful and evaluate your experience. When you quit on yourself and binge on food, you gain weight and feel a lot of food hangover pain. You also think more negative about yourself and feel more worthless, powerless, hopeless, and depressed. As a result, your urge to continue to binge on food to escape is stronger than ever and your motivation to pick yourself back up and try again is lower than ever.

NEVER SURRENDER

When it comes to failing, as long as you keep on picking yourself up afterwards, you can't lose. As the saying goes, "Winners never quit and quitters never win." Every time you fail, feel depressed, and hear your rock bottom reaction, be your own motivational coach and repeat to yourself over and over again that:

- You will never surrender.

- You will keep on fighting and learning.

- You can and will be successful.

- You are powerful.

When you have this mindset, even if you fail every day for weeks on end, you will still try to pick yourself back up every day and try again because you believe in yourself and know that quitting is not going to help—it's only going to make things worse. As you continue to fight after failing instead of quitting, you start to develop an inner resiliency. After a while, fighting and picking yourself back up becomes a habit/character trait and you end up valuing being resilient, and quitting no longer becomes an option. It's not something you will do no matter how down you are. You develop an attitude that you will keep on fighting until your last breath.

As long as you never give up on yourself and quit, you will never again lose yourself or gain lots of weight. This is how you can break your destructive eating habit of quitting and binging for days/ weeks after you fail.

CHAPTER 16:

CHANGING YOUR FOOD HANGOVER/PAIN EATING HABIT

THE FOOD HANGOVER

Whenever you make the value-choice to binge on food to escape, be mindful and feel the pain of your food hangover. You will feel symptoms like:

- Tiredness.

- Headache.

- Stomachache.

- Heartburn.

- Diarrhea.

- Dry mouth/throat.

- Irritableness.

As well, because you didn't make the rational, healthy value-choice, you experience negative feelings about yourself. All you feel like doing is binging on more food to escape the psychological, physical, and mental pain you feel. You tell yourself over and over how much pain you're in and how bad you feel.

Your automatic reaction to the feelings of pain caused by your food hangover, is to make self-defeating statements like:

- I can't and won't be able to follow my healthy living plan.

- I don't feel like cooking.

- I don't feel like exercising.

- I can't cope with the pain.

- I have to binge on food to escape.

After telling yourself the following and creating a self-fulfilling prophecy, more times than not, you convince yourself you have to binge on food to escape. Due to the pain you feel and how strong your desire to escape is, it does not take much negative self-talk to convince yourself to make that value-choice.

HOW TO COPE WITH PAIN

When you're feeling the painful effects of the food hangover, you have to take care of yourself and take it easy on yourself. When you're tired and in pain, it's harder to concentrate and focus your mind on your true, rational beliefs, and it's harder to muster up the energy needed to eat healthy and move your body. Your true, rational, and positive voice is weak and your false, irrational, and negative voice is strong.

Since you're already in a negative mood and don't feel like doing anything, it makes it more likely that you will give in to your urge to binge on food to escape. This is why when you're in this type of emotional state it's very important not to push yourself too hard. Any extra pressure and stress will just increase the pain and increase your urge to binge on food to escape.

A good first step to take when you're in pain is to be mindful and do some deep breathing exercises. Once you have achieved mind/body equilibrium and are no longer focused on the pain you feel, you can remind yourself of the rational truth. You can remind yourself that:

- You can follow your healthy living plan.

- You believe in the slow, steady, step-by-step, try-your-best approach.

- You don't have to be perfect.

- You believe in staying in the moment and being grateful for the day you've been given.

- You have the power and abilities to cope with the pain you feel.

When you feel more positive because your self-talk is more positive, be mindful and continue to make sure you're in control of your breathing. Focus all your attention on the moment and take one breath and one step at a time. For example, you could start by having a glass of water, making your bed, and taking a long, hot shower.

With every positive action and moment that passes, the better you will start to feel. One small positive action leads to the next and so on—until, you have made it through the day. When you're focused on an activity, it takes your mind off the pain, rather than sitting there dwelling on it. Which increases the pain you feel.

When you think to yourself that you can't make it through the entire day, remind yourself that you don't have to get through the whole day—you just have to get through the next second. Using this approach makes it easier for you to manage and control your strong urge to take flight and escape the pain. All you have control over is how you feel and act in the moment, so that is what you focus all your energy on. This is a more helpful strategy than taking on your whole day/life in the moment and stressing yourself out.

VALUE-COMPARISON

When you make the value-choice to react to the pain of eating too much by binging on even more food to escape, be mindful and take notice of how it only makes the pain more intense. Your headache will be stronger, your stomachache greater, your heartburn more intense, and you will feel sicker and more tired. It will now be harder for you to follow your true, rational beliefs and easier for you to follow your false, irrational beliefs and make the bad value-choice to binge on food to escape.

When you binge on food to escape the pain of your food hangover, you do escape the pain at first, but then you feel even greater pain later. What you have to ask yourself is if the short-term relief from pain is worth the long-term pain. Ask yourself how long the relief lasts and how long the pain lasts and do a cost-benefit analysis. What you find is that the price you have to pay for the short-term relief is way too high.

Now, when you are able to cope with your food hangover pain by calming yourself down and reminding yourself of the rational truth and end up following your true beliefs and making healthier choices, evaluate how you feel. What you will notice is that all your hangover symptoms lessen and your feelings of power and confidence increase.

Anytime you overcome pain, it makes you feel powerful. It provides you with proof that you are strong and can cope with some pain. This uplifts your spirit and motivates you to continue to try and do what you know is true and good, no matter how much pain you are in. By learning that you can cope with pain is how you can break your destructive eating habit of binging on food when you feel the ill effects of a food hangover.

CHANGING YOUR NO-BREAKFAST EATING HABIT

The best thing you can do after a day of overeating is to go right back to following your healthy living plan the next day. You're not going to feel like eating breakfast because you feel full, overweight, and are in pain, but you have to remind yourself that it's a very important part of being healthy and living healthy. This is why they have breakfast clubs at schools—it's to ensure each child feels calm and has the energy needed to focus their mind and learn. If they didn't eat breakfast, they wouldn't be able to pay attention while in class and would fall asleep or misbehave.

Breakfast is said to be the most important meal of the day. Having breakfast every morning will help you:

- Kick-start your metabolism.

- Make the next healthy eating choice.

- Focus mentally.

- Think rationally.

- Boost your mood.

- Boost your energy.

- Manage your hunger.

- Be more productive.

- Have a good start to the day.

When you learn for yourself that when you eat breakfast you feel better and perform better, you learn to value eating breakfast. You experience all of the above, which motivates you to want to eat breakfast.

What will also motivate you to eat breakfast is to be mindful of the negative consequences you experience when you don't. When you don't eat breakfast, pay attention to your energy levels, mood, and production. See if you end up eating unhealthy at lunch and are tired for the rest of the afternoon. If you ate a big lunch you probably won't eat again until your hunger is triggered later in the evening and you end up binging again. When you make the first bad choice to skip breakfast, it makes it easier to make the next one and so on.

By learning for yourself the pleasure and success you experience when you eat breakfast compared to the pain and failure you experience when you don't, is how you can break your destructive eating habit of skipping breakfast because you don't feel like it or don't have time. When you learn the value of it, you will make it a priority. For example, you will make sure you have healthy foods you can grab on the go like a banana and some peanuts/seeds.

There's an old saying, that if you want to avoid putting on weight, you should, "Eat breakfast like a king, lunch like a lord, and dinner like a pauper."

CHAPTER 17

CHANGING YOUR STRESS AND TOXIC G.A.A.S.S. EATING HABITS

HOW TO COPE WITH STRESS AND YOUR FIGHT-OR-FLIGHT RESPONSE

Once you have fought your way out of depression and rock bottom, you now have to cope with the stress caused by your value-conflict of wanting to eat healthy to lose weight, but also wanting to eat unhealthy to escape. This value-conflict creates inner stress as you fight with yourself to make the value-choice you know will help you achieve success and long-term pleasure, rather than the one you know will bring you immediate relief, but long-term pain later.

Every time you think about all the work you have to do and all the weight you have to lose, it creates extreme stress. Before, when you had to eat and exercise perfect to look perfect, the stress that these impossible expectations created was too much to cope with and you took flight and binged on food to escape. Your self-assessment was that in your current mental and emotional state, you were unable to meet these expectations. This is what triggered the flight response.

Now that you have changed your beliefs and learned some mind and body control techniques, you will be able to react differently to stress. Instead of taking flight, you will be able to stand up and fight.

The fight-or-flight response is intense and happens fast and before you know it you have taken flight and binged. It takes practice to be able to separate yourself from your strong reaction and be mindful. What will help is to become aware of the signs that you are under stress so you can change them. For example, when being mindful you will notice signs like:

- Your heart pounding.

- Your mind racing.

- Your stomach tightening.

- Your fists and teeth clenching.

- Your breath quickening.

When you focus in on your racing mind, you will hear extreme, conflicted, stress-inducing thoughts like:

- I need to binge and escape.

- I need to eat healthy and feel good.

- I need to lose weight.

- I can't take it.

- I have to binge to escape.

Whenever you find yourself in the battle between following your healthy living plan or binging on food to escape the stress you feel, do some deep breathing. Be mindful and focus on slowing down your breathing. When you slow down your breathing, you slow down all your other physiological reactions.

Once you're centred, calm, and back in control of your body and mind, refocus your mind on your true, rational beliefs and remind yourself that:

- You want to eat healthy and exercise because you love yourself.

- You believe in yourself.

- You no longer have to achieve the perfect body image.

- You don't have to win.

- You don't have to eat and exercise perfectly.

- All you have to do is take one moment and one step at a time.

- All you can do is try your best.

- Binging on food will not help you escape stress—it will only create more stress.

Once you are emotionally balanced and focused on your rational beliefs, you can then make healthier value-choices. By calming yourself down and repeating your true beliefs to yourself, you are able to de-stress and resolve your value-conflict peacefully. You then continue to just focus on your breathing, your true, rational beliefs, and taking one moment and one step at a time.

When you are able to successfully cope with your overwhelming stress and are able to successfully follow your healthy living plan instead of taking flight and binging on food to escape, you learn that you have the power to de-stress yourself and don't need to binge on food to escape stress. This knowledge increases your self-confidence and self-belief, which increases your motivation and determination to fight.

VALUE-COMPARISON

Now compare the above experience to when you make the value-choice to take flight from your stressful feelings and binge on food to escape. Whenever you make this value-choice—surprise, surprise—you end up feeling more stress. This is because you now have to cope with the pain of your food hangover and as you have learned this makes it even harder to follow your healthy living plan.

You are now not only stressed out, you're also in pain. Your value-conflict will be more intense because your desire to binge on food to escape will be stronger than ever. When you think about having to follow your healthy living plan feeling the way you do, it stresses you out because you don't feel like you can do it. This triggers your flight response where all you want to do is binge on food and escape.

By binging on food, you are able to escape stress temporarily. So again, you have to ask yourself if the short-term stress relief is worth the long-term, more intense stressful feelings and pain you will feel later. Of course, the true and rational answer is a resounding no!

When you learn the truth that by being mindful, doing deep breathing, and using CBT, you have the power to create true stress-relief, you can break your destructive eating habit of binging on food to escape stress.

CHANGING YOUR HABIT
OF BEATING YOURSELF UP
WHEN YOU FAIL

Once you're out of rock bottom and no longer quit after failing, you still have to learn how to cope with failure, so you don't feel the toxic G.A.A.S.S. feelings that also trigger your urge to binge and escape. Whenever you fail to follow your healthy living plan, your automatic, destructive emotional reaction is to become angry and beat yourself up and call yourself negative names.

It's the emotion of anger over failing to achieve something you wanted, that starts your toxic reaction. It's easy to tell when you're angry because you're usually jumping around and cursing loudly. If not that, your blood is boiling, your heart is pounding, and your fist and teeth are clenched. When you pay attention to your mind, you will hear yourself say things like:

- I can't believe it.

- I'm pissed.

- Curse this and curse that.

- You idiot, you jerk.

As you continue to "trash-talk" yourself, you go through the rest of the toxic emotions. Guilt is the next emotion you usually feel. When you feel guilty, you feel remorse and feel like punishing yourself. You know you're feeling the emotion of guilt when you hear yourself saying things like:

- I shouldn't have.

- I wish I didn't do it.

- How could I?

- I'm bad.

After guilt comes anxiety. Anxiety creates a strong physiological and physical response. For example, your heart pounds, your stomach tightens, your temperature rises, and you breathe faster and you pace. This is accompanied by a racing mind filled with anxious thoughts like:

- I'm in trouble.
- I'm doomed.
- What's going to happen?
- I don't know what to do.

The last two emotions you go through are shame and sadness. Shame makes you feel embarrassed and you can feel yourself "turning red." You feel like hiding yourself away. These feelings of embarrassment are caused by thoughts like:

- I'm so overweight.
- I'm not normal.
- Other people must think negative about me.
- I don't want to be seen.

Lastly, you feel sad. When you feel sad, you feel down. Your physiological and physical responses, like your mood, is low. The same goes for your thinking. By being mindful, you will hear yourself repeating statements like:

- I always fail.
- Nothing works out for me.
- It's not fair.
- I'll never be successful and happy.

These are the toxic thoughts and evaluations that are running through your head as you beat yourself up for failing. Your mind goes back and forth between the past mistake you made and your doom-and-gloom overweight future. This attack on yourself and life makes you feel the toxic G.A.A.S.S. emotions that trigger you to want to binge on food to escape. Just like you have been doing, you have to fight your destructive feelings and urges by calming yourself down and refocusing your mind on your true, rational beliefs.

When you are being mindful and notice (by becoming aware

of physiological and physical reactions) that you are feeling toxic G.A.A.S.S. after failing, start by doing some deep breathing. Again, this is so you can slow down your reaction and regain control over your body and mind. Once calm and back in control of your faculties, focus on your mind and challenge your false and toxic thinking with your true, rational beliefs and remind yourself that:

- You forgive yourself.

- You love yourself.

- You believe in yourself.

- You will never quit.

- You believe that losing weight is not easy.

- You believe in your plan and approach.

- You're blessed.

- You're not perfect and that's okay.

- You're learning new knowledge and skills, and that making mistakes is part of the process and part of being human.

When you remind yourself of your true, rational beliefs, your feelings of toxic G.A.A.S.S. are replaced with feelings of self-worth, self-confidence, hope, and happiness. The rational truth of who you are and why you're trying to eat healthy, is what makes you feel better, which in turn makes you want to pick yourself back up and try again. As the Buddha said, "Anger will never disappear so long as thoughts of resentment are cherished in the mind. Anger will disappear just as soon as thoughts of resentment are forgotten."

ONWARD AND UPWARD

Instead of kicking yourself when you're down, you learn that you have to encourage yourself and pick yourself up after failing. You have to remain positive and confident in the face of failure and frustration. It's a natural reaction to feel down when you try hard and still lose, but you have to learn that "crying over spilled milk" and "raking yourself over the coals" after failing does not help and is, in fact, self-defeating. When you're telling yourself you're a failure and you're focused on your past failures, chances are you're going to fail again.

You have to learn that you can't change the past or control the future—all you can do is focus your mind on the moment and try to do better. To be successful in the future, you have to be able to let go of your past failures and negative feelings. For example, if a goalie in any sport lets in a goal they should have saved, they have to be able to let it go so they can focus all their power and abilities on making the next save. If they remain upset about the mistake or are worried about making another mistake, it increases the likelihood they will let in another soft goal.

The most important thing you need to do when you fail is to learn from your mistakes and move on. In order to be successful, you have to go through the process of failing and learning. You have to learn why you failed, to learn what not to do the next time. This is how you learn what it takes to be successful.

Since failing is part of learning, if you don't learn how to cope with failing, you will never be successful. Remember, life is not about winning or losing—it's about learning. When you make errors (and you will), be a kind, patient, encouraging teacher to yourself. Rather than telling yourself you failed, tell yourself you learned and move on.

VALUE-COMPARISON

Now, be mindful and pay attention to what happens when you beat yourself up after failing and react to your toxic G.A.A.S.S. feelings by binging on food. When you do, you will find that you feel more intense toxic G.A.A.S.S. later. This is because you end up feeling even worse about yourself.

You become an emotional wreck as you go through the process of feeling each toxic emotion more intensely. Your mind is filled with negative self-evaluations and your body is full of intense, negative emotions, which makes it harder for you to calm yourself down and focus your mind on your true, rational beliefs and easier for you to react to your strong urge to binge on food to escape. You also feel the painful effects of the food hangover, which further increases your urge to binge.

Once again, you are able to escape the toxic G.A.A.S.S. and pain temporarily when you binge on food, so you have to ask yourself if the short-term relief is worth the long-term pain. Reflect on how long the relief lasted and how long the pain lasted. I know you know what the true, rational answer is.

By going through this process of feeling the intense, toxic G.A.A.S.S. emotions and toxic food hangover pain every time you binge after beating yourself up for failing, is how you can break this destructive emotional eating habit. Just like going through the process of feeling better and eating better every time you encourage yourself after failing, is how you learn that encouraging yourself is a better way to cope with failing.

CHANGING YOUR WIN-OR-LOSE EATING HABIT

When you no longer have to follow an unrealistic diet program to achieve the perfect body image in order to feel good about who you are, you no longer have to win. When you don't have to win to feel good about yourself, there is no losing yourself. You might not be happy with yourself when you overeat, but you no longer lose your self-worth, self-confidence, and quit on yourself.

Now if you eat unhealthy during the day, instead of thinking that you have lost and feeling bad about yourself and concluding that you now might as well eat bad for the rest of the day, you continue to follow your eating plan, or at the very least try your best to eat as healthy as possible. For example, just because you ate a hamburger and fries for lunch does not mean you now have to have pizza for dinner. You could instead have a healthy cooked meal and a piece of fruit for dessert.

When you eat something that was not on your plan, all you have done is made one bad choice and ate some extra food—you haven't lost anything. The next time you eat, you have the chance to reassert your power by making the value-choice to follow your healthy eating plan. By repeating this behaviour of eating a healthy meal after eating an unhealthy meal, is how you can break your win-or-lose eating habit.

CHANGING YOUR PRESSURE AND PLEASURE EATING HABITS

HOW TO COPE WITH PRESSURE

Whenever you live healthier and lose some weight, you start to feel better. As soon as you feel good, you are confronted by your desire to eat for pleasure rather than your desire to eat to escape pain. As discussed in the relapse stage, when you fight your cravings, you feel the pressure of your value-conflict of wanting to follow your diet plan and lose weight, but also wanting to binge on food to feel pleasure.

When you're under pressure, you feel some of the same physiological and physical symptoms you feel when you're under stress (although less intense). By paying attention to your body, you will feel your heart beating faster, your breath quickening, and your body tightening. By paying attention to your mind, you will hear yourself saying contradictory thoughts like:

- I want to eat.

- It will be good.

- It will be fun.

- A little won't hurt.

- I deserve it.

- I can't eat.

- I have to lose weight.

- I have to win.

- I can't win.

- I can't do it.

- I can't take the pressure.

- I have to binge on food to escape.

Just like you calmed yourself down when you were feeling stress, focus on controlling your breathing. Do some deep breathing until your body is relaxed, and you're centred and balanced. Then, challenge your false, irrational self-talk with the rational truth and remind yourself that:

- You accept and love yourself as is.
- You don't have to lose weight.
- You don't have to win.
- You believe you can do anything.
- You believe in the slow, steady, step-by-step, try-your-best approach.
- You believe your healthy eating plan provides full satisfaction and pleasure.
- You don't have to eat, but can if you really want to.

When you are able to relieve yourself from the pressure and are able to continue to follow your healthy living plan, you learn that you don't have to "white knuckle" it. You learn that by using the powers of your mind, you can rationally talk yourself through the pressure instead of willing yourself through it. Using willpower only lasts for so long before you burn out and give in to your urge to relieve yourself from the constant pressure you feel.

Once again, you learn the valuable lesson that you can relieve yourself from your intense feelings and resolve your value-conflicts peacefully by controlling your breathing and by controlling your mind. This adds to your already growing self-worth, self-confidence, hope, and happiness.

VALUE-COMPARISON

When you make the value-choice to eat to escape pressure, evaluate your experience. Yes, you escape the pressure in the short-term, but you feel even more in the long-term. Since you're in more pain and gained more weight, you now put even more pressure on yourself to follow your plan. As well, since you gave in to your urge to eat to escape, it's that much stronger. This makes the value-conflict more intense and more difficult to resolve, but of course, not impossible.

You now know how to cope with the pressure and resolve your conflict peacefully by calming yourself down, reminding yourself of the rational truth, and taking one step and one moment at a time. You will then be in the right mental and emotional state to be able to make the true, good value-choice to follow your healthy living plan. This is how you can break your destructive eating habit of bingeing on food to escape pressure.

HOW TO COPE WITH YOUR CRAVINGS

Not every time you feel your cravings do you fight them and feel the pressure of your value-conflict. Sometimes you give in to your cravings right away. Whether your cravings are triggered by the time of day or by the sights and smells of food at home or in your social environment, you will want to have some.

The unhealthy food you love and crave is everywhere and available anytime. As well, every month there seems to be some celebration or holiday that involves lots of unhealthy food and drinks. For example, for almost the entire month of December your cravings will be triggered by all the food and drinks that will be offered to you for free. It's a tough month for anyone trying to eat healthy.

Cravings are very powerful and can trigger you to act immediately. For example, picture Homer from the television show, *The Simpsons*, when he is triggered by seeing or thinking about donuts and goes into a trance-like state and floats towards his object of desire. To be able to stop yourself from reacting automatically to your cravings, you have to learn to recognize the signs of being triggered. When you're able to do this, you can stop yourself before you automatically satisfy your cravings.

By being mindful, you can learn to recognize the signs that you have been triggered by a craving. Here are some of the physiological, physical, and mental signs that you're being triggered by your urge to eat for pleasure:

- Faster breathing.

- Flared nostrils.

- Mouth watering/Licking of lips.

- Intense visual and mental focus on the foods of your desire.

- Repeating to yourself over and over how hungry you are and how good it will be.

- Automatic movement toward the object of your desire.

There is a passage from the Bhagavad Gita (The Hindu Bible) that brilliantly captures what happens to you when you're triggered by something desirable: "When a man dwells on the pleasures of sense, attraction for them arises in him. From attraction arises desire, the lust of possession, and this leads to passion, to anger. From passion comes confusion of mind, then loss of remembrance, the forgetting of duty. From this loss comes the ruin of reason, and the ruin of reason leads man to destruction."[64]

When you're triggered by your desires, you temporarily lose your rational mind. When this is lost, you forget about your rational beliefs and values and lose self-control. This is when you act on your impulse and feelings, and usually end up regretting it afterwards.

Since cravings are so strong and all it takes is a split second to act on an impulse, you have to be mindful. When you're mindful and feel in your body that you're being triggered by a craving, and hear yourself trying to talk yourself into binging on food, go back to focusing on slowing down your breathing. Do some deep breathing exercises and when your body and mind has slowed down, use CBT to challenge your cravings with the rational truth. Remind yourself that:

- Your healthy eating plan is not a restrictive diet.

- You can eat more if you want, but you're choosing not to.

- The short-term pleasure is not worth the long-term mental, physical, and psychological pain you will feel.

- You're trying to feel better.

- You're not hungry.

- It will be harder to follow your healthy living plan later.

- You love yourself.

- You believe in yourself.

- You are thankful for all you have and don't need more.

Once you're refocused on the rational truth and feel better, you're better able to make the value-choice to follow your healthy living plan. As long as you don't immediately react to your cravings and take a moment to breathe and think about the truth, your cravings will weaken and your rational, true voice becomes stronger.

Every time you're able to outsmart your strong cravings, and instead follow your healthy living plan, the stronger you feel. You feel stronger, because you have proven to yourself you have the power to cope with your powerful cravings and can do what you know is true and good. As result, your self-confidence and trust in yourself to do what you say you're going to do, grows exponentially.

VALUE-COMPARISON

When you do give in to your cravings and "reward" yourself, evaluate your experience. Ask yourself if satisfying your cravings really did bring you pleasure, and if so, was it worth the long-term pain? You have to find out for yourself if eating what you like is a reward or a punishment?

We all know how pleasurable eating certain foods can be, but the pain you feel afterwards can leave you wondering if it's worth it. When you eat too much of the food you love, you feel the food hangover pain along with your toxic G.A.A.S.S. feelings. This means you have to spend the rest of the day, and/or the next day, feeling negativity and pain. As well, every time you give in to a craving the stronger it becomes and the harder it is to deny. Whether it's wanting to escape pain or satisfy a craving, both feelings make it more difficult to focus on the rational truth and follow your healthy eating plan.

If you go through this process of rationally and critically evaluating your experience every time you eat for pleasure, you learn for yourself that in the end, all you experience is pain. You start to see that every time you do eat for pleasure, you don't feel or perform your best afterwards. Since you love yourself and want to feel and do good, you will make every effort to avoid the pain caused by so-called pleasure eating. To be able to resist satisfying your constant cravings, you have to learn for yourself that the short-term gratification is just not worth the long-term pain you will feel later.

Only when you have learned that you hate the feelings caused by eating unhealthy, more than you love to eat unhealthy, will you be able to fight your urge to eat for pleasure. This is because only a learned rational and conscious value has the power to fight a natural or conditioned value. This is how you can break your destructive pleasure eating habit.

CHANGING YOUR ALL-OR-NOTHING EATING HABIT

When you no longer value food as a source of pleasure (as much), you also change your destructive all-or-nothing eating habit. This is the habit where you eat as much of the food you love as you can before you start your next diet. Which is usually on a Monday. This is because Monday represents a fresh start, a new week, and a new beginning. For example, if you decide on Friday you're going to start a new diet on Monday, you proceed to eat as much of the unhealthy food you love as possible. This is due to the fact that you know once you start your diet, you will not be able to have these foods.

As discussed previously, when you eat unhealthy and feel negativity and pain, your urge to eat to escape increases—which decreases your chances of success. This is why more times than not you ended up failing to follow your diet on the Monday.

By being mindful and analyzing your experiences, you now know that you're not denying yourself anything except pain when you choose not to binge on food for pleasure or relief. As a result, after a "diet fail" more time than not you'll go back to following your healthy eating plan later in the day, or at worse, the next day.

What also makes you go back to following your healthy eating plan is that your diet is not restrictive, and it includes a lot of foods you like. This is how you can break your all-or-nothing eating habit.

CHANGING YOUR NIGHT-TIME EATING HABIT

Whether it's eating to escape stress or pain, or eating for pleasure, my strongest urge to eat, hits me at night time. When I used to be triggered to binge before bed I would go back and forth in my head, fighting and trying to decide if I should eat or not. As you have learned, this just increases the pressure and stress you feel, which increases your urge to escape. You reach the point where you feel you have no choice, but to eat if you want to calm yourself down enough to be able to fall asleep.

This is how the night-time eating habit is formed.

I now play fewer head games with myself. I know what is true and good, and I know what to do. I'm not going to let my destructive emotional eating habits talk me into eating, when I rationally know it will only cause me pain. So as soon as I feel the physical and physiological reactions caused by pressure/stress or cravings, I focus in on slowing down my breathing to relax my body, quiet my mind, and balance my emotions. This stops my reaction and gives me the time to regain control and talk rationally and truthfully to myself. I then remind myself of my true, rational beliefs and I remind myself of the consequences of my value-choices.

I tell myself that if I don't eat, I will:

- Be in a good mood when I wake up.
- Feel powerful for having resolved the conflict peacefully and constructively.
- Have lots of energy.
- Be able to focus and think rationally and critically.
- Feel good physically.
- Feel like eating breakfast and following my healthy living plan.

If I do eat, I will:

- Be in a negative mood when I wake up.
- Feel less powerful because I resolved the value-conflict destructively by giving in to my emotions and urges.
- Have low energy.
- Be more mentally unfocused, irrational, and emotional.
- Feel overweight and physically ill.
- Not feel like eating breakfast and following my healthy living plan.

Reminding myself of the true consequences of my behaviour helps me make the value-choice to follow my true beliefs and healthy living plan. I have learned from experience that the long-term negative and painful consequences associated with night-time eating, is not worth the short-term relief or pleasure.

VISUALIZATION

I also find it helpful to use the mental technique called visualization. This involves mentally playing the movie in your head about what your day will look like if you choose to eat late and what it will look like if you don't. I envision having to go through the day feeling like crap and having to interact with other people and be productive while in a negative and painful emotional state. I will then envision myself making the right value-choice and waking up feeling good and having a good day. This is usually enough for me to make the value-choice to not eat and just go to sleep.

RETURN TO YOUR ROUTINE

When I do eat at night, I wake up the next day, have breakfast, and continue to follow my healthy living plan. Even though I might not feel like having breakfast, I know this is what will make me feel better and what will help get me back on track.

VALUE-COMPARISON

Since I like to eat at night so much and it does at times help me fall asleep (not sleep well), it wasn't until I went through the process of re-evaluating my night-time eating habit that I learned it's not worth it. I had to feel the pain over and over of waking up not feeling good and having a crummy day before I began to no longer value it. I had to learn for myself that it does not help me escape pain or feel pleasure; it only causes me long-term pain. Only when I learned the rational truth did I have the power to consistently fight and change my late-night eating urges. This is how you too can break a destructive night-time eating habit.

CHANGING YOUR BINGE-EATING HABIT AND THE VALUE OF YOUR MIND

Going through each one of your destructive emotional eating habits and evaluating your experience is how you learn the truth that binging on food, whether it's to escape pain or satisfy cravings, does not work and only brings long-term pain. You will have felt the pain of being stuffed and sad over and over and will have proved to yourself that it's not worth it. As a result, you will no longer value binging (as much) as a way of eating to escape pain or feel pleasure.

As well, because you now know how to resolve your value-conflicts and cope with your emotions and cravings, there is less of an urge to binge. Your emotions and cravings no longer build up to an intense level where you feel like you have no choice but to eat. When you're calm, in control, and have a plan, there is no need to binge.

Again, because you're only human, when you do decide you're going to make the value-choice to not stick to your healthy eating plan and are going to eat food to escape pain or satisfy pleasure, tell yourself that you will do the least harm to yourself that you can. Instead of binge eating, you can do what I call harm-reduction eating.

HARM-REDUCTION EATING

Harm-reduction is a treatment method used to help people that have serious addiction issues, but are not ready or willing to go cold turkey. For example, for people who inject drugs, the goal is to ensure that they have access to clean needles, so they don't become infected with a disease. For alcoholics, the goal is to ensure they drink actual alcohol, so they don't drink the more harmful cooking wine or rubbing alcohol.

The goal for people who struggle with food follows somewhat the same philosophy. Unlike drugs or alcohol, you cannot go cold turkey with eating. You have to eat to live. This is what makes curbing a food dependency/addiction a challenging task.

Also, we live in an environment filled with unhealthy food (and stress) that is available and marketed 24/7—meaning your urge to binge will be triggered on a daily basis. You are bound to give in to your emotions and urges every once and a while, and this is where using a method like harm-reduction can be very helpful.

Using the harm-reduction technique means that when you do "decide" to eat to escape pain or satisfy a craving, you try to eat the "healthiest" unhealthy food you can find and try to have the smallest amount of it you can, while still feeling pleasure or pain-relief. For example, instead of eating ice cream, you could have yogurt or cereal; instead of chips you could have trail-mix; and instead of regular chocolate you could have dark chocolate. The more natural the ingredients are, the less triggered you are to binge.

Today, there are more junk food and processed food products on the market that have less saturated fat, trans fat, sugar, and salt, and still taste good. Again, this is why it's so important to read those labels. There are certain foods I no longer eat, like pastries; after becoming aware of the high amounts of fat and sugar they contain.

You can save yourself a lot of extra fat, sugar, salt, weight, and pain when you use harm-reduction eating. When you engage in this type of eating, sometimes you don't even have a food hangover. By using harm-reduction eating, you can still satisfy your desire to eat while lessening the mental, physical, and psychological pain.

The next day, even if you feel some pain and are upset, you have to acknowledge the good you did do. At least you showed some self-control and made some good choices. You have to remind yourself how much worse it could have been. This makes you feel better and encourages you to keep on trying to follow your plan and fight through the pain.

You can also use harm-reduction eating when you eat out. For example, ask for whole grain carbs, put sauces on the side, and make healthy substitutions like a salad instead of fries. If you have fast-food, have a small drink instead of a super-large and if you're at a BBQ have the hamburger without the processed cheese.

When cooking or baking you can substitute certain ingredients. For instance, you can use cinnamon instead of sugar, and avocado instead of mayonnaise. Be creative and have fun. Food is supposed to be healthy, and healthy food is supposed to taste good.

FEED THE BEAST

The worst thing you can do is deny your cravings, because they will only become stronger. When you wait until the breaking point to satisfy them, you end up binging. This is what causes you the extra pain and the extra weight.

It's always better to attack a craving before it attacks you. Most times it's better to eat some than trying to eat none. When you satisfy your urges to eat on your terms (not due to being triggered) you decrease your chances of engaging in binge eating. Since you're not emotional when you eat, there is no need to binge. As a result, your urge to eat can be satisfied by having a little, rather than needing a lot.

This is why it's important to include healthy snacks that you like in your daily meal plan. As long as you're eating foods you enjoy on a frequent basis, your cravings are rarely triggered. It's all about you managing and being in control of yourself and your life.

VALUE-COMPARISON

If you end up eating more than you wanted to (since that's what a lot of junk/processed food is designed to make you do), be mindful and feel the pain. It's by being mindful and feeling the negative and painful consequences of binging on food to escape pain or feel pleasure over and over that you can break your destructive binge-eating habit.

Being mindful and feeling the less damaging effects of harm-reduction eating over and over is also how you replace binge eating with the less painful and destructive harm-reduction eating.

THE VALUE OF YOUR MIND AND THE RATIONAL TRUTH

Once you have gone through the long process of breaking all of the destructive emotional eating habits you developed, you break your dependency on using food to cope with your emotions and cravings. You will now depend on yourself and your own mental coping powers. Just like you no longer focus on external fast and easy diet programs to lose weight and your external body to feel worthy, powerful, hopeful, and happy, you no longer focus on external food to bring you pleasure or pain-relief. You now look to your internal self and focus on your powerful mind and your rational true beliefs.

By rationally and critically evaluating your experiences, you will have learned for yourself that reacting emotionally and binging on food does not help you escape pain or bring you pleasure—it only brings you long-term pain. Instead, you will have learned that:

- By being mindful, doing deep breathing exercises, and using CBT, you have the power to control your feelings, thoughts, and behaviour.

- By re-focusing your mind on your true, rational beliefs you have the power to make yourself feel good and do good.

- Your mind is the most valuable and powerful part of who you are.

Now, being mindful, doing deep breathing exercises, and using CBT to remind yourself of your true, rational beliefs, becomes the way you cope with your destructive emotional reactions and destructive urges to eat. You will have experienced for yourself that this method of coping brings you greater pain relief and greater pleasure than binging on food ever did. This makes you value your new way of coping. As a result, being mindful and rational becomes a value-priority and the focus of your attention. When this happens, being mindful and rational becomes your *modus operandi* and you're better able to remain in control and change your destructive emotional reactions and urges. Which allows you to make the rational value-choice to follow your healthy approach and healthy living plan.

What will also help you follow your new approach and new plan is to learn that by doing so, you experience great pleasure and great pain relief. You already know how painful it feels to eat and live unhealthy; now you have to learn how good it feels to eat healthy and exercise. In order to follow your new approach and new healthy lifestyle for the long-term, you have to learn to value/like it.

CHAPTER 20 :

LEARNING HOW TO VALUE YOUR NEW APPROACH AND NEW HEALTHY LIVING PLAN

RESOLVING YOUR LIFESTYLE CONFLICT

Due to your past negative experience, your automatic, conditioned, emotional reaction is to not like to eat healthy and exercise. As previously discussed in the success stage, eating healthy and exercising was seen as the price you had to pay to lose weight. This is why you stopped doing it once you lost weight and went back to living the way you like, which was to eat unhealthy and not exercise. Until you learn to value eating healthy and exercising, you won't continue to do it once you have lost weight.

As a result of following diet and exercise programs, you never learned how to eat healthy and exercise. You were either on an extreme, restrictive, rigid, demanding, unrealistic diet and exercise program or you were binging on food and not exercising. It's time for you to learn how to eat healthy and exercise in a rational and realistic way.

Learning how to truly eat healthy and exercise is how you learn that eating healthy and exercising is a reward that brings pleasure and is not a punishment that causes pain. You have to learn that it brings you greater pain-relief and greater pleasure than eating unhealthy and not exercising ever did. When you learn this, you will want to eat healthy and exercise for the rest of your life.

A good example of someone who learned this truth is the comedienne/actress Rosie O'Donnell. She was on the Dr. Oz show talking about the heart attack she had and said that eating junk food almost killed her and that now it no longer has the pull on her that it used to. She went on to say that if anyone told her that she would like and enjoy eating healthy she would not have believed it. This highlights the importance of having to learn the truth for yourself.

When you learn firsthand that using your new rational approach to living healthy brings you pleasure and not doing it brings you pain, it motivates you to want to do it. This is how you resolve your internal value-conflict of having to follow your healthy living plan, but not wanting to or not feeling like it. Now when you're in the internal battle to follow your plan or not, you can remind yourself not only of the pain you will feel if you don't do it, but of the pleasure you will miss out on if you don't. You can tell yourself that it will help make you feel better.

To learn this truth for yourself, you need to be mindful and focus your attention on how you feel when you make the value-choice to use the slow, steady, step-by-step, try-your-best approach to eat healthy and exercise. Every time you do, ask yourself, "How do I feel mentally and physically? How do I feel about myself? How productive was I? Was the short-term struggle, worth the long-term pleasure?"

Being mindful and asking yourself these questions is how you will become aware of all the inner rewards you experience when you use your new approach to eat healthy and exercise. This is what will change your evaluation regarding eating healthy and exercising from negative to positive.

When you learn the truth about eating healthy and exercising, you will learn that you have been denying yourself by making the value-choice to not do it. Instead of craving food, you should be craving to eat healthy and exercise because it makes you feel so good. I'm sure you have heard some people say that exercising can be addictive and that runners experience a high. This is how you can exchange a bad habit that brings short-term pleasure with a good habit that brings long-term pleasure.

Let's first take a look at what you experience when you make the value-choice to use your new approach to eat healthily.

HEALTHY EATING:
COMPASSIONATE EATING

Right from the start, because you're using the slow, steady, step-by-step, try-your-best approach, you will notice that you're in a calmer state rather than feeling stressed-out. This is because you no longer have to perfectly follow a restrictive diet or achieve the perfect body image and lose X amount of weight in X amount of days. Your reason for trying to eat a healthier diet is to feel good because you love and care about yourself. All you're focused on is making one, two, or even a few changes to your eating plan. It's up to you to experiment and figure out what you can reasonably and realistically handle.

DISCIPLINED EATING

One of the first couple of changes I recommend you make is eating breakfast and then eating every 3-4 hours afterward. The goal should be to eat three meals (breakfast, lunch, and supper) and two snacks, with at least one of those meals being all-natural.

The first thing you will become aware of when you eat this way is that you have more energy and feel more positive throughout the day. This makes you feel more mentally alert and more emotionally calm, which improves your ability to focus your mind on making good, rational choices. This is the opposite of feeling tired, lethargic, irritable, irrational, and making emotional choices. As people say, now you won't be "hangry" (meaning you're angry because you're hungry).

Also, by starting your day off with breakfast it sets you up for having a structured, disciplined day. For example, by making the choice to eat breakfast it increases the chances that you'll eat lunch and so on. Everything flows in its natural order.

If you don't eat breakfast in the morning, then you will be having breakfast when you should be having lunch, and lunch when you should be having dinner. Your whole schedule is out of whack and you end up having to play catch-up for the rest of the day. This makes your day more stressful, which increases your chance of binging.

Eating at regular times also reduces impulse eating. Again, because you're eating every few hours or so there is less opportunity for impulse eating. For example, if you happen to be triggered by a craving before your scheduled time to eat, you know you won't have to wait long.

As well, when you skip meals your blood sugar and energy levels drop, which triggers your urge to binge. For instance, if you skip breakfast you increase your chances of being hungry and eating a lot at lunch. Just like if you don't plan for a snack after lunch and come home hungry, you increase your chances of eating a lot at dinner. It also increases the likelihood you will choose the processed/junk food that you desire and can have fast and easy. Since your hunger is triggered, you want to eat immediately and not in ten or fifteen minutes.

Pay special attention to how positive and powerful you feel, when you always feel satisfied and in control of yourself and your eating. You will see that following a balanced diet leads to balanced emotions and a balanced day. Jenny Mayhem, poetically posted this in a response to an article on how to diet effectively: "Self-discipline is a reward in itself! There is so much more satisfaction in a day of truly healthful eating than there is at the bottom of a bag of chips."[65]

It makes you feel powerful and confident and less confused and anxious when you know what and when you're eating. You don't have to waste time debating or wondering (as you try to make up your mind) about what you're going to eat—you already know. It's one less thing you have to worry about, which lessens your stress, which lessens your urge to binge. As a wise person said, "only a disciplined mind can bring you happiness."

It also feels good to follow your healthy eating plan and check things off your to do list. You feel like a well-oiled machine, which makes you feel productive and powerful. This proves to yourself that you can achieve your goals and do what you say you're going to do—which, increases your confidence and trust in yourself and your abilities.

NO NIGHT-TIME EATING

Eating healthy and at regular times also helps you to sleep more soundly. Any healthy eating plan should include not eating three (give or take an hour) hours before bedtime. Be mindful and pay attention to both how much better you sleep and how much better you feel when you wake up. For example, you will have less heartburn and indigestion, you will toss around less, and you will feel more refreshed when you wake up. This increases your mental abilities and motivation to follow your healthy eating plan.

A good night's sleep is known to help people manage their weight, just like not sleeping well is known to help you gain weight. One study stated that people who don't get enough sleep are less likely to prepare their own meals and are more likely to depend on restaurants and fast-food establishments for some of their meals.[66] Since you're tired and you're in a negative emotional state, you're more likely to react impulsively and eat food you can have fast and easy. As Dr. Mike Evans said in an article about how sleeping too little or too much can lead to weight gain, "When you're tired and run down, you're just not making the great life decisions."[67]

MINDFUL EATING

When you do eat a healthy meal, be mindful and pay attention to how much slower you eat, and how quickly you feel full. By being mindful when you eat, you can become aware of how small your stomach is and how small healthy meals make you feel satisfied. As my mother always said to me when I wanted a lot of food and couldn't finish it, "your eyes are bigger than your stomach."

Compare this experience to when you eat unhealthy food and eat fast and it takes forever to feel full. Humans are triggered to eat as much fatty, salty and sugary food when given the chance. The mechanism that signals you're full—is turned off. You don't stop until you're stuffed and in pain.

If you notice yourself eating fast, you know your urge to binge has been triggered and you should stop eating and do some deep breathing. When you're calm and in control, go back to eating slowly and mindfully.

When you feel even slightly full, stop eating. You don't want to eat until you're entirely full. By eating small meals throughout the day, you never have to feel the pain of being stuffed again.

NATURAL EATING

In addition, when you eat healthy pay attention to how good it tastes. Eating healthy is supposed to taste good. Natural food, cooked simply and seasoned lightly, brings out its natural flavors. This is what chefs like Jamie Oliver's food revolution is trying to teach people. He is going across North America showing people that natural food is not hard to prepare and tastes great.

We have become so used to eating foods with saturated/trans fat, sugar, and salt, we have forgotten what natural food tastes like. For example, vegetables can be eaten naturally without butter and salt, and whole grain cereal can be eaten without sugar. Over time, you will become so used to eating so-called plain, real food that when you eat food with too much salt or sugar, you will find it repulsive.

If you haven't eaten natural food for a while, you have to give your taste-buds time to adapt. You will learn to like the taste, just like you will learn to like eating heathy for all the reasons stated above.

Now let's take a look at what happens when you make the value-choice to use your new approach to exercise.

HEALTHY EXERCISING: COMPASSIONATE EXERCISING

Again, because of the approach you're using, you will feel calmer and will be focused on healing and feeling good. This is because you no longer have to worry about exercising for X amount of minutes, or lifting X amount of weight to achieve the perfect body image in X amount of weeks. Your reason for exercising has changed. You now do it because you love yourself and want to take care of yourself. All you're focused on is moving your body in a way that makes you feel joy.

MINDFUL EXERCISING

When you exercise, be mindful and pay attention to how good you feel mentally, psychologically, and physically. Observe how good it feels to be moving your body.

When you're doing cardio, visualize and feel your heart beating, your lungs breathing, your blood pumping, and your body parts moving. Focus on controlling your breathing as you inhale in and exhale out. For example, one, two, three in and one, two, three out.

When you're lifting weights, do it in a slow and controlled manner and visualize and feel the muscles you're working out. To ensure you are using all your muscles equally to lift the weights, it can help to visualize your weaker side working. Focus on controlling your breathing as you inhale in and exhale out.

Here's what writer Sibylle Preuschat had to say about the benefits of mindful motion: "Of course, any physical exercise – walking, swimming, yoga – is good for your brain, too, but to up the mental empowerment quotient pay attention to what you're doing muscle by muscle. Focusing establishes new neural pathways that can help sharpen the mind into old age and improve your ability to learn, remember and function."[68]

TRANSFORMATIVE EXERCISING

Notice that when your mind and body are working in harmony you feel at one with yourself and the universe. Besides the endorphin rush, you feel this way because you're doing something you were built to do.

Humans have been walking, running, jumping and lifting since inception—all things we did to survive and thrive as a species. As well, it's all things we did as children to play and have fun. When you're moving your body, you feel alive and happy.

By moving your body, you also burn off pent-up pressure and toxic emotions, and are able to de-stress and re-set. While you're exercising, you're able to quiet your mind and let your body take over for a while. Since you're able to shut off your mind and focus on your body movements, it gives your mind a break from your problems and all the internal chitter chatter.

Focus on how good it feels when your mind is quiet, your body is relaxed, and your emotions are calm. It brings you feelings of peace, harmony, and balance. As Jenny Rumancik, author of the book *I Met Jesus At The Gym* stated in an interview on 100 Huntley Street, "I love just the feeling of being at the gym and walking and listening to your worship music and just having that quiet time to work on yourself and your physical and emotional state."

INSIGHTFUL EXERCISING

As a result of your mind being focused on moving your body, exercising is a great time for "a ha" moments. Answers to questions and problems you have been working on solving will come to you in flashes of profound insight. This is because when you are mentally quiet (stopped your self-talk) and your emotions are calm, you are better able to hear the wisdom that lies within your own brain.

DISCIPLINED EXERCISING

By exercising at the time you said and by doing what you know is the best thing for your health adds to your feelings of self-control and self-power. Exercising not only strengthens your heart, lungs, bones, and muscles, it also strengthens your self-confidence. It adds further proof that you can trust yourself to do what you know is true and good.

What you will also discover is that following your exercise plan provides further structure to your day. The more structure you have, the less impulsive you are. As the saying goes, idle hands is the devil's playground. Again, focus on how good and empowering it feels to know what you're doing and when you're doing it.

Exercising, also motivates you to follow your eating plan. You don't want to do something good for yourself and then do something bad for yourself.

SELF-ENHANCEMENT EXERCISING

Your self-confidence is further boosted when you see yourself improving. Exercising offers a tangible experience where you can see yourself growing and getting better. For example, if you can exercise a bit longer or lift a bit more weight, you can see yourself incrementally making progress. It can give you something to work on and work towards.

As well, pay attention to how much more motivation and energy you have. When you exercise regularly, you feel like you can do anything and you have more passion for life. You engage in life more and your performance is better in everything you do. Exercising gives you that little extra pep in your step. Plain and simple, you have a better, happier, and more productive day when you exercise.

When people say they don't have the energy to exercise, what they have to realize is that the reason they don't have energy is because they're not exercising. This point cannot be emphasized enough. Exercising gives you energy.

NATURE EXERCISING

I really recommend that when ever possible, you exercise outdoors. When you do this, you receive double the benefits. Not only do you feel the healing effects of moving your body, you also feel the healing effects of nature. Seeing the blue sky, feeling the warm sun, and breathing in fresh air induces positive, healing emotions.

If you can, exercise by or in water. The healing powers of water, whether seeing, hearing, or feeling it, is known to every human. This is why a lot of people sing in the shower or take a long, hot bath.

PEACEFUL EXERCISING

When you're finished exercising, be mindful and focus on how refreshed, reenergized, and relaxed you feel. Pay attention to how good this feels.

Also, notice that when you encounter pressure, stress, conflict, or disappointment, you're in a better mental and emotional state to deal with it in a rational and productive manner. You will see that you don't react as strongly or at all. This is because you're in a calm and centred state and not an emotional state. As you have been learning, when you're more emotional, you're more easily triggered to react emotionally and irrationally.

Lastly, when it's time to sleep, because you're calm and relaxed from burning up all your negative energy, take notice of how you fall asleep easier and have a deeper, peaceful sleep. When you wake up, you'll find that you have more energy and a more positive attitude as you start your day.

THE VALUE OF LIVING A HEALTHY LIFESTYLE

After going through this process of rationally and critically evaluating your experience when you make the value-choice to follow your new approach and new healthy living plan, you will have proven to yourself that it brings you great pain-relief and great feelings of pleasure and power. You will have experienced the calmness and the boosts to your energy, happiness, confidence, and performance. This is the opposite of what you experienced when you followed the perfect, fast, and easy diet and exercise approach.

Instead of feeling conflict, intense emotions, and cravings when you try to eat healthy and exercise, you feel inner peace, calmness, and satisfaction. You will have learned that you don't need to eat like a "prisoner" or exercise like a "commando" to achieve health benefits. Rather, eating and exercising mindfully and moderately leads to greater health and greater enjoyment.

You now know that if you want to feel better than okay you have to make eating heathy and exercising a part of your daily life. If you don't do these two things, you know you won't be at your best and won't have as good a day as you could have.

Even though you rationally know all of this, there will still be times you won't want to do it. Every time you have planned to eat healthy or exercise, and hear yourself say, "I don't feel like it," do some deep breathing exercises and remind yourself that:

- There is no more pleasurable or powerful feeling than being in control of yourself and your actions.

- There is no more pleasurable and powerful feeling than making the value-choices that you rationally know bring you success and happiness.

- Having a peace of mind (due to resolving value-conflicts rationally and constructively) is more pleasurable than having a piece of cake.

- All you have to do is take it slow, take one step-at-a time, and try your best.

- Living the healthy life is living the "perfect life."

By reminding yourself of these truths, it increases the chances you will make the value-choice to follow your healthy living plan. You have to ask yourself why you would want to deny yourself the opportunity to feel pleasure and power.

Once you value eating healthy and exercising, you will make following your healthy living plan a priority. This means for eating, you will:

- Create a meal plan.

- Go shopping so you have the food you need for the week.

- Pack the food you need for the day to ensure you're able to eat every three hours.

- Cook at least one all-natural meal a day.

When it comes to exercising, you will:

- Create an exercise plan.

- Set aside the time.

- Incorporate it into your daily life.

- Invest in the proper gear and equipment.

When you really learn to like living heathy, you might even start buying recipe and nutrition books and exercise magazines to learn more. There are whole industries built around eating healthy and exercising. For example, for jogging, there are the shoes, the outfits, the water bottles, and the tech gadgets. There are even running clubs and marathons you can be part of. Depending on how deep you go, exercising can become a major part of both your fashion style and life-style.

For eating healthy, there are cooking classes and an endless number of blogs and websites. There is also a new food movement where people who want to eat natural go to local farmers' markets and shop at special health food stores. They only buy and eat locally grown, organic food. It's often tied into being green and environmentally friendly. How far you go all depends on how much you value it.

TRUE PATH AND PURPOSE

When you learn the true value of your mind, your beliefs, your approach, and your healthy living plan, is when you learn the true answers to your last two rock bottom questions, "How can I lose weight?" and "What is my purpose?"

By learning that you can control and change your destructive emotional reactions and destructive emotional eating habits using mindfulness, deep breathing, CBT, the rational truth, and the slow, steady, step-by-step, try-your-best approach, they become your new values and your new answer to how you can lose weight. You will have experienced for yourself that this is the true path to long-term self-worth, self-confidence, hope, happiness, and weight management.

Once you learn what your true path to success and happiness is, you learn the answer to your last rock bottom question, "What is my purpose?" Before, your answer was having to lose weight so you could achieve the perfect body image and live live the perfect, "skinny," happy life. After learning what is true and valuable, your purpose changes to having to control your inner mind and body so you can control your destructive emotional reactions and urges and live the "perfect," healthy, happy life. You now know your focus needs to be on controlling your emotional and irrational self if you want to be able to follow your true beliefs and live the healthy lifestyle that brings you true feelings of pleasure and power. This purpose is reflected in a line from The Native American Prayer by Yellow Hawk – Sioux chief, "I seek strength not to be superior to my brothers, but to be able to fight my greatest enemy, myself."

Knowing your true path and purpose becomes especially important once you have lots of success and lose lots of weight. Every time you have lost weight before and reached the success stage, you eventually gained it back plus more. Now that you have learned the rational truth and changed your belief and value system, the next time you reach the success stage, you will be able to stay there.

CHAPTER 21

LEARNING HOW TO MAINTAIN WEIGHT LOSS SUCCESS

HOW TO COPE WITH WINNING

When you have broken all of your destructive emotional eating habits, have been following your healthy living plan every day, have lost a lot of weight, and have regained your full self-worth, self-confidence, hope, and happiness, is the exact moment you have to be most careful and most mindful. You are at your most vulnerable when you're having success and feeling good. In a journal article about relapse prevention, it had this to say about this stage: "The final and most important stage of the change process is the maintenance stage. It is during the maintenance stage (which begins the moment after the initiation of abstinence or control) that the individual must work the hardest to maintain the commitment to change over time. It is during this stage that the person will be faced with a plethora of temptations, stressors, and the pull of powerful old habit patterns."[69]

It's easy to become caught up in the excitement of losing weight. You feel fantastic, you look fantastic, and family, friends, and even strangers are complimenting you on your appearance. This makes it easy for your focus to change to how you look and wanting to celebrate your weight loss success.

Before, living the perfect, "skinny," happy life was seen as the reward for all your sweat, struggle, and sacrifice. After all the pain you went through to lose weight, it was now your time to experience the pleasure of being "normal" and "fitting-in." Once your focus changed to your appearance and being socially successful, it was not long before you went back to living the way you love, which was to eat unhealthy and not exercise.

You were now being driven by your feelings of pleasure rather than by your feelings of pain. All you focused on was experiencing pleasure and having fun without thinking about the consequences. This is because you wanted to feel pleasure and not the pain of denying yourself. You already did enough of that. You told yourself that you deserved to treat yourself and that a little extra food and missing an exercise session here or there wouldn't hurt.

You falsely believed you had everything under control and would never gain weight again. Since you had just lost weight and were feeling great about yourself, you thought you were invincible. As you have learned, missing a few and having a little turned in to a lot and without you realizing it, you were no longer in the habit of following your diet and exercise program, and were gaining weight and losing yourself. You were unaware you were relapsing, and on your way back to rock bottom.

Since you are now aware of who you are and what is true and valuable, and know how to cope with your triggers and destructive self-talk, this time you will be ready for success.

SET UP FOR LONG-TERM SUCCESS: TRUE SELF

First of all, since you have accepted, loved, and believed in yourself when you were overweight and have been counting your blessings along the journey, when you lose weight there is no big spike in your feelings of self-worth, self-confidence, hope, and happiness. There is no intense state of euphoria or excitement. You do feel good about yourself that you have succeeded at losing weight, but not because of how you look, but rather because you fought to follow your true, rational beliefs and made good value-choices. You now know that this is where true, positive, and powerful feelings of self come from.

You have learned who you are and will no longer lose your true self because you lost lots of weight. Your self-image is no longer dependent on your body image. You are now more dependent on yourself and your valuable, powerful mind. Since you are more focused on the rational truth, you are more grounded in reality and are not carried away by your feelings of pleasure and power due to your weight loss. As a result, your focus remains on your inner self to feel good about yourself, instead of on your fleeting outer appearance.

TRUE PLEASURE

Secondly, because you have learned for yourself that there is no greater pleasure than following your healthy living plan, you want to do it all the time. As a result, there is no desire to quit living healthy after weight loss success. This is because you have been enjoying yourself and feeling good every time you eat healthy and exercise. You have been eating foods you like and moving the way you like, so you don't feel like you have been denying or forcing yourself to do anything.

On the flip side, since you have learned that eating unhealthy and not exercising brings you pain, this is the last thing you want to do. Whether it's the weekend or a special holiday, you will try to stick to your plan as much as possible because you now know nothing else allows you to enjoy your day more fully and be more successful at everything you do. You will have experienced for yourself that living healthy is the reward and that eating unhealthy and not exercising is the punishment.

When you do decide to indulge in some unhealthy food and drinks (and again you will, because you're only human) you will be motivated to use the harm-reduction technique and will return to your healthy living routine immediately. You do this (more times than not), because you love yourself and want to feel pleasure, not pain.

You also try to make the rational, good value-choices because you are now too keenly aware of how one bad value-choice can lead to more bad value-choices and to more pain. Before you know it, you're back in the habit of binging on food to escape pain. You have to remind yourself how strong your destructive emotional reactions and urges are and how easily they can take over your mind and body—which makes it hard for you to think and act rationally. Remember, it takes only a few weeks to replace a good habit with a bad habit. Then, you will have to fight twice as hard and as long to break it.

TRUE PATH AND PURPOSE

Lastly, you have learned that if you want to continue to follow your rational beliefs and continue to make the rational, healthy value-choices that make you feel positive and powerful, you have to continue to be mindful and focus your attention on your inner mind and body. You are now aware that it takes less than a second to act on an irrational thought or destructive urge and that the only way you can stop yourself and change your destructive emotional behaviour is to be self-aware. This is why being self-aware of your inner mind and body becomes your new priority.

No matter whether you're feeling pain or feeling great, you have to make sure you're being mindful and that your body is relaxed, your emotions are balanced, and your mind is focused on the rational truth. This is how you will continue to follow your new, true, rational belief and value system no matter how you feel.

DAILY MIND RESET

Unlike reacting emotionally and irrationally, being mindful so you can ensure you are thinking rationally and critically is not an automatic behaviour. It's a conscious, intentional behaviour. This means, every single day you have to consciously choose to make it your number one priority and the focus of your attention.

It takes effort and hard work to be mindful. We lose our focus and attention easily. Our concentration is broken by both our mind's thoughts and our senses. This is why you have to always remind yourself to be mindful and rational.

Being mindful takes daily practice. You have to take your time and take it easy on yourself. It's natural and easy to become caught up in your thoughts and feelings, and all the things you have to do in life. The next thing you know the day is over and you were not able to be mindful.

If you forget to be mindful one day, at least you are aware of it and try again the next day. With practice, slowly you will become more mindful until it becomes a strong habit.

If you are having trouble being mindful during the day, you could be mindful before bed. For example, an hour before bed you could check in with your inner state and if your mind is racing and you're feeling anxious or stressed, you could do some deep breathing to calm yourself down and quiet your mind.

You can also try to be mindful in the morning. If you start doing it first thing, hopefully you will continue to do it for the rest of the day.

What can also help is to set your alarm to beep every ten minutes to remind youself to be mindful about your inner state.

By being mindful on a daily basis, you will never again have another "Oh no" moment and gain a lot of weight without you noticing. Your self-awareness allows you to catch yourself when you see yourself falling back into old, destructive behaviour patterns. You have to remain diligent and vigilant. When it comes to controlling your old, false, destructive beliefs, values, and behaviours, you can never let down your guard. This is what makes managing your weight a lifetime endeavour.

If ever you should find yourself struggling and lose your way, you now know the path back home. You now know the way back is to go within and be mindful, breathe, challenge your self-talk, focus on the rational truth, and use the slow, steady, step-by-step, try-your-best approach to ease yourself back into the habit of eating healthy and exercising.

Good luck on your inner journey of self-discovery, self-understanding, and self-happiness!

APPENDICES

APPENDIX 1 (a):
HOW MANY CALORIES

When it comes to setting up your own healthy eating plan, one of the big questions is, "How many calories should I eat?" When it comes to calories, you have to decide what number you feel good at. If you listen to other people, you will be left confused.

How many calories "experts" say you should eat is all over the map. It ranges from 1200-2200 calories for the average woman and from 1500-2700 calories for the average man.

By 2018 the Ontario Government in Canada is making certain food establishments put on their menus that: "Adults and youth (ages 13 and older) need an average of 2000 calories a day, and children (ages 4 to 12) need an average of 1500 calories a day. However, individuals needs vary."

Which amount of calories is right for you? How many calories is too low, how many calories is too high? What is your Goldilocks amount? To find this out you have to ask yourself, at what calorie amount do you feel healthy and have the energy to fulfill your daily demands? You have to experiment with different caloric intakes and see how you feel. If you're feeling light-headed, have a headache, and have no energy, you're eating too few calories. If you're feeling stuffed and lethargic, you're eating too many calories. When you feel healthy and have the energy to function at a high level, you're eating the right amount of calories for you.

CALORIE-COUNTERS

You can go on the internet and use websites that provide calorie-counters. All you have to do is punch in your gender, age, weight, height and activity level and the amount of calories you should eat a day to maintain your current weight will be calculated.

There are now also apps that will calculate how many calories you should eat given your particulars.

CALORIE CHARTS

You can also use charts that will show you how many calories a person for your gender, age, and activity level should eat as a guideline but again, you are the best person to decide how many calories you should eat. Below is a calorie chart that comes from Canada's Food Guide that you can use as a guide to assist you in estimating how many calories you should eat a day. This chart can be found at: www.healthcanada. gc.ca/foodguide.

ESTIMATED ENERGY REQUIREMENTS

Males (Calories per day)

Age	Sedentary 1 Level	Low Active 2 Level	Active 3 Level
2 - 3 y	1000	1350	1500
4 - 5 y	1250	1450	1650
6 - 7 y	1400	1600	1800
8 - 9 y	1500	1750	2000
10 - 11 y	1700	2000	2300
12 - 13 y	1900	2250	2600
14 - 16 y	2300	2700	3100
17 - 18 y	2450	2900	3300
19 - 30 y	2500	2700	3000
31 - 50 y	2350	2600	2900
51 - 70 y	2150	2350	2650
71 y+	2000	2200	2500

1   Sedentary: Your typical daily routine requires little physical movement (e.g., sitting for long periods, using a computer, relying primarily on motorized transportation) and you accumulate little physical activity in your leisure time.

2   Low Active: Your typical daily routine involves some physical activity (e.g., walking to bus, mowing the lawn, shoveling snow) and you accumulate some additional physical activity in your leisure time.

3   Active: Your typical daily tasks involve some physical activity and you accumulate at least 2 ½ hours of moderate- to vigorous- intensity aerobic physical activity each week. Moderate- to vigorous- physical activity will make you breathe harder and your heart beat faster.

Females (Calories per day)

Age	Sedentary 1 Level	Low Active 2 Level	Active 3 Level
2 - 3 y	1100	1250	1400
4 - 5 y	1200	1350	1500
6 - 7 y	1300	1500	1700
8 - 9 y	1400	1600	1850
10 - 11 y	1500	1800	2050
12 - 13 y	1700	2000	2250
14 - 16 y	1750	2100	2350
17 - 18 y	1750	2100	2400
19 - 30 y	1900	2100	2350
31 - 50 y	1800	2000	2250
51 - 70 y	1650	1850	2100
71 y+	1550	1750	2000

1   Sedentary: Your typical daily routine requires little physical movement (e.g., sitting for long periods, using a computer, relying primarily on motorized transportation) and you accumulate little physical activity in your leisure time.

2   Low Active: Your typical daily routine involves some physical activity (e.g., walking to bus, mowing the lawn, shovelling snow) and you accumulate some additional physical activity in your leisure time.

3   Active: Your typical daily tasks involve some physical activity and you accumulate at least 2 ½ hours of moderate- to vigorous- intensity aerobic physical activity each week. Moderate- to vigorous- physical activity will make you breathe harder and your heart beat faster.

These values are approximations calculated using Canadian median heights and weights that were derived from the median normal BMI for different levels of physical activity.

Your individual values may be different. The requirement for energy varies between individuals due to factors such as genetics, body size and body composition. These values are not for women who are pregnant or breastfeeding.

To approximate your individual estimated energy requirement, use the information provided.

WEIGHT SCALES

Another way of trying to figure out if you're eating the right amount of calories is to weigh yourself. If you're gaining weight, you're eating too much. If you're losing more then 1 to 2 pounds a week, you're eating too little. If you're losing no weight at all, you're eating enough to maintain your weight. If you want to lose weight, you're either going to have to decrease your caloric intake, increase your activity level, or do a little of both.

APPENDIX 1 (b):
CALORIES IN, CALORIES OUT

To maintain your weight, the number of calories you consume has to be equal to the amount of calories you burn, or else you will likely gain weight. The problem is that it's not that easy to determine exactly how many calories you burn in a day. This is because as your body performs such functions as breathing, digesting, and regulating your temperature, you burn calories. For example, even when you watch television or read a book, you burn anywhere from 80-100 calories per hour depending on your gender and body type.[70]

An article stated that the average 150-pound person burns about 1800 calories a day just in the act of living.[71] So, if the average 150-pound person did any exercising or engaged in any extra activities, the amount of calories they burned would be more. For example, if they go for a jog and burn 200 calories, they would have burned 2000 calories for the day. This means they would need to eat 2000 calories to maintain their weight.

There are 3500 calories in one pound of weight. So, if they wanted to lose one pound a week, they would have to burn approximately 500 calories more than their consuming a day. Using the example above of burning 2000 calories a day, to lose one pound a week, they would have to consume 1500 calories a day and that would give them the 500 calorie a day deficit.

COUNTING CALORIES

You might not know exactly how many calories you burn a day, but you can know approximately how many calories you eat a day. For every food you eat, the calorie amount can be found by searching on the internet. As well, all processed foods you buy in the grocery store list the serving size and the calorie amount on their packaging. All you have to do is list all the foods (and amounts) you ate (or are going to eat) in a given day and add up the total calories. You can then adjust accordingly.

APPENDIX 2:
SERVING SIZES

Serving sizes is as important as the types of food you eat. Even if you eat too much healthy food, you will not feel good and you will gain weight. This list of what is considered to be one serving size comes from Health Canada's Food Guide.

PROTEIN:

- Cooked fish, shellfish, poultry, lean meat: 75 g (2 ½ oz.)/125 mL (half cup)
- 2 eggs
- Shelled nuts and seeds: 60mL (quarter cup)
- Peanut or nut butters: 30 mL (2 tbsp)
- Tofu: 150 g or 175 mL (¾ cup)
- Cooked legumes: 175 mL (¾ cup)

DAIRY:

Milk or powdered milk (reconstituted): 250 mL (1 cup)

Canned milk (evaporated): 125 mL (½ cup)

Fortified soy beverage: 250 mL (1 cup)

Cheese: 50 g (1 ½ ounces)

Yogurt: 175 g (¾ cup)

Kefir: 175 g (¾ cup)

STARCHES:

Bread: 1 slice (35 g)

Bagel: ½ bagel (45 g)

Flat breads: ½ pita or ½ tortilla (35 g)

Cooked rice, bulgur, or quinoa: 125 mL (½ cup)

Cooked pasta or couscous: 125 mL (½ cup)

Cereal: cold: 30 g and hot: 175 mL (¾ cup)

VEGETABLES:

Fresh, frozen, or canned vegetables: 125 mL (½ cup)

Leafy vegetables: cooked 125 mL (½ cup) and raw 250 mL (1 cup)

FRUIT:

Fresh, frozen, or canned fruit: 1 fruit or 125 mL (½ cup)

100% Juice: 125 mL (½ cup)

OIL and FATS

Cooking oil, salad dressings, butter, and mayonnaise: 30 to 45 mL (2 to 3 Tbsp) of unsaturated fat each day.

RECOMMENDED AMOUNT OF SERVINGS FOR EACH FOOD GROUP

The Canada Food Guide recommends servings per day based on your age and gender. The serving sizes per day are smaller for the young and larger for the old. Here is a range of what is recommended for each food group. If you want the full list, it's available on-line at: www. healthcanada.gc.ca/foodguide.

Vegetables and Fruit: 4 to 10

Grain: 3 to 8

Milk and Alternatives: 2 to 4

Meat and Alternatives: 1 to 3

Some of the numbers seem too high to me and I don't eat as many servings as they recommend, especially the number for grains, and vegetables and fruit. These are just recommendations and a guide, so use it as such. Again, you are the one that can best determine what the healthy and correct amount is for you based on your tastes, lifestyle, and budget.

APPENDIX 3 (a):
NUTRITIONAL LABELS

For your own health and well-being, you need to know the nutritional content of the food you are consuming. You should know as much as you can about the make-up of the food you are eating and how much of it you are eating so you can ensure you are eating the recommended nutritional amounts. More and more this information is becoming available. Now it's up to you to start to use your rational and critical thinking powers to analyze it.

SERVING SIZE

When reading the nutritional facts you have to pay particular attention to the serving size. This is what the nutrition amounts are based on. Look to see if the information is based on the box, one cup, or even less. If the nutritional information is based on a small serving size and you know you eat double that, you have to multiply all the nutrients by two to know how much you will be eating. For example, if you're buying ice cream and the label is based on a ¼ cup and you know you will have a cup, you have to multiple the amounts by four to know how much fat and sugar you will be eating.

Setting up a menu plan based on the daily recommended nutrient amounts will help ensure you are eating a balanced, healthy diet. You have to make sure the amount of calories you need to eat are aligned with the amount of nutrients you need. For example, if you are eating the recommended daily amount of fat, sugar, and sodium in half the calories you need, you will have to make healthier food-choices.

DAILY PERECENTAGE VALUES

The daily percentage values listed on the label for each nutrient is based on an average daily intake of 2000 calories. This information can help you see the approximate daily percentage value of each nutrient you are eating per serving. For example, the fibre could be 7g per serving which would represent 28% of the daily recommended amount.

APPENDIX 3 (b):
RECOMMENDED NUTRIENT AMOUNTS

Here is a list of the daily recommended amounts of fat, sodium, sugar, fibre, carbohydrates, and protein you should aim to eat. Again, there is no magic number. The numbers are all over the place and how they came up with the numbers is not scientifically stated. These numbers are meant to be used as guides to see if you are at least in the "ball park" with the numbers you are eating.

PROTEIN:

A 150-pound person needs 69 grams of protein. You can use this as a guideline depending on your gender, age, weight, and activity level.

If you try to aim for around 20 g of protein at each meal you can't go too far wrong. For example, 3 oz piece of chicken has 26g, a 3 oz piece of wild salmon has 21g and one cup of black beans has 15 g of protein.

It's also been recommended that 30% of your total caloric intake should come from protein.

FAT:

If you're eating a healthy diet, you will be consuming mostly natural, healthy fats and less of the saturated fats. It's recommended you consume no more than 20 grams of saturated fat and eat as little trans fat as possible.

The American Heart Association recommends that just one per cent of an individual's total calories should be from trans fat.[72] It was said that for a 2000 calorie diet, that's just two grams of trans fat daily, or about half a bag of small fries.[73]

The Heart and Stroke Foundation recommends that 20 to 35 per cent of the calories a person eats a day should come from fat.[74] It stated that for an average female on a 2000 calorie diet, that would equal 45 to 75 grams of fat a day.[75] For an average male on a 2500 calorie diet, that would equal 60 to 105 grams of fat a day.[76]

SODIUM:

When it comes to salt, the recommend intake is[77]:

1000 mg for children aged 1-3
1200 mg for children aged 4-8
1500 mg for people aged 9-50
1300 mg for adults aged 51-70

The Heart and Stroke Foundation of Canada suggests Canadian adults eat no more than five millilitres of salt (2300 milligrams of sodium or a teaspoon of salt) per day.[78] Consuming 2300 milligrams of salt is the tolerable level, whereas 1500 is the more adequate level.[79] It's been stated that for your body to function under normal circumstances, it needs only 500 mg of sodium a day.[80]

Sodium is especially high in processed foods, so it's important to read those labels. Even food you think is healthy could be high in sodium. In an article about bread topping the list of salt sources in the U.S. diet it stated: "For example, a slice of white bread can have between 80 and 230 milligrams of sodium. One cup of canned chicken noodle soup has between 100 and 940 milligrams. And 3 ounces of luncheon meat has between 450 and 1,050 milligrams."[81]

SUGAR:

The American Heart Association guidelines for added sugars are:

26 grams or 9 teaspoons for males
20 grams or 5 teaspoons for females
12 grams or 3 teaspoons for children

Try to stick to the single digit rule. For example, if you're buying cereal purchase a product that has less than 10 grams per 1 cup. Even though this will not be easy to find, there are some no sugar and no sodium cereals on the market.

CARBOHYDRATES:

There are carbohydrates in almost every food you eat, so it's hard to measure. It's recommended that you eat between 200 to 325 grams of carbohydrates a day. Try to aim for the lower end of the range if your caloric intake is around 1800 calories.

FIBRE:

The daily recommended fibre intake ranges from 25 to 38 grams.

APPENDIX 4:
STARTER EATING AND EXERCISE PLAN

Remember to always consult with your physician before starting any new diet and exercise plan.

MENU PLANNING

You have to decide if you're going to set up a seven day plan and repeat it at the end of the week or if you need a shorter plan. I suggest you try and keep what you eat as simple as possible. The goal is to not create too much stress with the changes you are making. For example, you could set up a three day program to begin with. This will make it easier to keep track of what and how much you are eating. As well, when you go grocery shopping you won't have to pick up too many different items or plan and cook many different meals.

A SAMPLE THREE DAY EATING PLAN

Here is a sample of what your meal plan could look like for the day.

Breakfast: Serving of milk and cereal, rice cake with serving of peanut butter and a banana.

Lunch: Tuna on whole wheat pita with raw carrots and celery on the side and an apple for dessert.

Snack: Protein bar and serving of seeds/nuts.

Dinner: Serving of chicken with a serving of couscous and veggies, and a kiwi for dessert.

Snack: Serving of berries wth a serving of natural yogurt.

Keep everything else the same except for dinner and have, for example, salmon, rice, and veggies one night and lentils with potatoes and veggies the next night and then repeat. You could also switch up the protein you put in your pita.

A SAMPLE TWO DAY EXERCISE PLAN

CARDIO: Choose one day and go for a 20 to 30 minute brisk walk/ jog. This can be done indoors by running on the spot and/or lifting your knees and moving your arms. This is in addition to incorporating more movement into your daily life.

STRENGTH-TRAINING:

Choose one day to do a full body workout which will take 20 to 30 minutes.

To start off, all you will need is a set of dumbbells that range from two pounds to fifteen pounds. Even if you're really strong, you won't need dumbbells higher than twenty-five pounds in the beginning. It's actually better to use lighter weights when you're learning how to do a new movement. You can control your movements better and focus more on your form to ensure you're doing the exercise correct and are working out the correct muscles. If you begin with heavy weights before learning how to do a movement properly, you could pull or strain a muscle.

The exercise examples provided for each major muscle group can be found on the internet. I recommend you do a search or look in some fitness magazines on how to properly and safely perform these and other exercises before trying. As well, you can join a gym and hire a personal trainer to help guide you in the beginning.

I suggest you start with one set for each exercise and aim for eight to twelve reps. When you are able to do this comfortably, you can do two sets and can even go up to three sets.

Once you start to strength train more than once a week, you can split up the muscle groups you workout. For example, one day you could workout your chest, shoulders, legs, and triceps and on the other day, your back, biceps, and abs.

EXERCISES

CHEST: Standing Chest Press - 1 set of 8-12 reps

SHOULDERS: Standing Military Press - 1 set of 8 to 12 reps

ARMS: Dumbbell Bicep Curls - 1 set of 8 to 12 reps
Dumbbell Tricep Extension - 1 set of 8 to 12 reps

BACK: One-Arm Dumbbell Row - 1 set of 8 to 12 reps

LEGS/LOWER BODY: Squats – 1 set of 10 to 15 reps

STOMACH: Basic Crunch - 1 set of as many as you can do.

NOTES

1. "Your View: What experiences have you had with weight loss products,?" CBC News, Last Modified February 17, 2009, www. cbc.ca

2. "Eating disorder awareness week," National Eating Disorder Information Centre, 200 Elizabeth St., ES 7-421, Toronto, Ontario, M5G 2C4, Canada, (copyright NEDIC 2003).

3. Ibid.

4. Ibid.

5. "Worsening obesity epidemic calls for new approach," CBC News, Last Modified Oct 4, 2011, www.cbc.ca

6. "Doctors call for weight loss industry regulation," CBC News, Last Modified February 17, 2009, www.cbc.ca

7. "Does dieting make you fat,?" CBC News, Last Modified April 13, 2007, www.cbc.ca

8. Dr. Bret Taylor, "Self-absorption just isn't good for you," CBC News, Last Modified April 30, 2008, www.cbc.ca

9. Laura Cummings, "The Diet Business: Banking on Failure," BBC News, Last Modified February 5, 2003, www.news.bbc.co.uk

10. "Does dieting make you fat,?" CBC News, Last Modified April 13, 2007, www.cbc.ca

11. Ibid.

12. Ibid.

13. "EATING DISORDER AWARENESS WEEK," National Eating Disorder Information Centre, 200 Elizabeth St., ES 7-421, Toronto, Ontario, M5G 2C4, Canada, (copyright NEDIC 2003).

14. Steven Van Beek, "You can do it," Now Magazine, October 4-10, 2007, p.37.

15. "Doctors call for weight loss industry regulation," CBC News, Last Modified February 17, 2009, www.cbc.ca

16. Ashley Montagu, Man: His First Million Years (New York:The New American Library of World Literature, Inc.,1958), p.15.

17. Nathaniel Branden, The Psychology of Self-Esteem (New York: Bantam Books, Inc.,1969), p113.

18. Peter Hadzipetros, "Eating to numb the pain," CBC News, Last Modified August 30, 2007, www.cbc.ca

19. John W. Santrock, Steven R. Yussen, Child Development Fifth Edition (Iowa: Wm. C. Brown Publishers, 1992), p.68.

20. Santrock, Yussen, p.68.

21. Chuck Gallozzi, "Balancing self-improvement with self-acceptance," Outreach, July 25-May 1, 2003, p.3.

22. Kaleb Montgomery, "Don't sweat your splurge," Now Magazine, December 30, 2004-January 5, 2005, p.31.

23. Cathrine Moller, p.31.

24. Pamela M. Peeke, "Stress Makeover," Prevention, September 2001, p.111.

25. Stephen P. Robbins, Nancy Langton, Organizational Behavior (New Jersey: Prentice-Hall, 1999), p.159-162.

26. G. N. Molloy, Et Al., "Locus of control of smokers, nonsmokers, and non-practising smokers," Psychological Reports, vol. 81(1997): p.781-782.

27. Willow Lawson, "Are you overweight? Depressed? The two problems may be linked," Psychology Today, Last Modified June 9, 2016, www.psychologytoday.com

28. Steven Reinberg, "Obesity and depression often twin ills, study finds," Health Day News, Last Modified October 16, 2014, www. health.usnews.com

29. "Why people attempt suicide," NHS Choices, Last Modified September 9,2016, www.nhs.uk

30. Health Behavior News Service, "Body image tied to suicidal thoughts in young teens," Wise, Last Modified August 29, 2013, www.newswise.com

31. Ibid.

32. "Wentworth Miller: 'I was suicidal'," 24 Hours, March 30, 2016, p.13.

33. Ibid.

34. "Stressed is just desserts spelled backwards," CBC News, Last Modified February 10, 2009, www.cbc.ca

35. "The Bellwood Eating Disorders Recovery Program," Bellwood Health Service, 1020 McNicol Avenue, Scarborough, Ontario, M1W 2J6.

36. David D. Burns, M.D., Feeling Good (New York: Penguin Group, 1981), P.11.

37. Adria Vasil, "Inuit author Sheila Watt-Cloutier takes the moral high ground in her mission to save the Arctic," Now Magazine, April16-22, 2015, p.24.

38. Chuck Gallozzi, "Balancing self-improvement with self-acceptance," Outreach, July 25-May 1, 2003, p.3.

39. Alvin and Virginia B. Silverstein, Exploring The Brain (New Jersey: Prentice-Hall, 1973), p.13.

40. Joel Thuma, "Six steps to a healthy heart," Healthy Directions, February/March 2005, p.8.

41. Joan Borysenko, Ph.D., Minding the body, mending the mind (New York: A Bantam Book/published by arrangement with Addison-Wesley Publishing Company Inc., 1988), p.147.

42. Andrew Roberts, Et Al., Creativity Course Kit – Second Edition (North York: York University, 1995), p.iv.

43. Chuck Gallozzi, "Many live lives too small for their spirits," Outreach, May 27-June 3, 2005, p.3.

44. Ashley Montagu, Man: His First Million Years (New York: The New American Library of World Literature, Inc., 1958), p.13.

45. Chuck Gallozzi, "Responsibility is not a burden, it's a blessing," Outreach, May 30-June 6, 2003, p.3.

46. Abdul-Rehman Malik, "Awareness of death makes life more precious," The Toronto Star, August 26, 2000.

47. "Canadians have no time for healthy living," CBC News, Last Modified November 29, 2011, www.cbc.ca

48. "Sudden, extreme exercise risks damaging kidneys," CBC News, Last Modified January 13, 2013, www.cbc.ca

49. "Bit of exercise helps overweight women improve fitness: study," CBC New, Last Modified May 15, 2007, www.cbc.ca

50. Mayoclinic.com, Mayo Clinic, www.health.msn.com

51. Psychology Today.com, Psychology Today, www.health.msn.com

52. Mayoclinic.com, Mayo Clinic, www.health.msn.com

53. Ibid.

54. Tara Weiss (Forbes.com), "Staying healthy and fit when your job is going or gone," CBC News, Last Modified February 16, 2009, www.cbc.ca

55. CBC Market Place, "Temptation abounds," CBC News, Broadcast October 29,2002, www.cbc.ca

56. Andrea Holwegner, "Good nutrition isn't all bad," CBC News, Last Modified April 16, 2008, www.cbc.ca

57. Mayoclinic.com, Mayo Clinic, www.health.msn.com

58. Dr. Lance Levy, Conquering Obesity (Toronto: Key Porter Books Limited, 1951), p.71.

59. Ibid., p.63.

60. H. Gunaratana Mahathera, "Mindfulness In Plain English," Buddhasasana, Last Modfied January 29, 2005, www.saigon.com

61. Ibid., p.10

62. Dennis Greenberger & Christine A. Padesky, Mind over mood (New York: Guildford Publications, Inc., 1995), p.v.

63. Thich Nhat Hanh, Peace of mind (California: Parallax Press, 2013), p.12.

64. The Bhagavad Gita (Middlesex: Penguin Group, 1962), p.54.

65. Rebecca Ruiz, Forbes.com, "Is your diet passe?" CBC News, Last Modified February 16, 2009, www.cbc.ca

66. "Health benefits of sleep," CBC News, Last Modified February 22, 2011, www.cbc.ca

67. "Sleeping a little, or a lot, can lead to weight gain, researchers find," CBC News, Last Modified, April 1, 2008, www.cbc.ca

68. Sibylle Preuschat, "Mind your motion," Now Magazine, June 10-16, 2004, p.40.

69. G. Alan Marlatt, Relapse prevention: Theoretical rationale and overview of the model, p.1.

70. Fred Rohe, The complete book of natural foods (Colorado: Shambhala Publications, INC., 1983), p.125.

71. "Diets: A primer," CBC News, Last Modified May 17, 2004, www.cbc.ca

72. "Trans fats: The move away from bad fats," CBC News, Last Modified July 21, 2008, www.cbc.ca

73. Ibid.

74. Ibid.

75. Ibid.

76. Ibid.

77. "Nutrition: How much sodium do I need?," CBC News, Last Modified July 26, 2011, www.cbc.ca

78. The Associated Press, "Bread tops list of salt sources in U.S. diet," CBC News, Last Modified February 8, 2012, www.cbc.ca

79. "Nutrition: How much sodium do I need?," CBC News, Last Modified July 26, 2011, www.cbc.ca

80. Ibid.

81. The Associated Press, "Bread tops lists of salt sources in U.S. diet, CBC News, Last Modified February 8, 2012, www.cbc.ca

I would really like to hear from you regarding your thoughts about the book.

Please email me at:
davidpaulpowell@rogers.com

PLEASE SUBMIT A SHORT REVIEW OF MY BOOK ON THE PRODUCT DETAIL PAGE AT: www.amazon.com

JOIN ME ON FACEBOOK/
David Paul Powell

AND

VIEW MY YOUTUBE CHANNEL/
David Paul Powell

To learn about my weight management services, please visit:
www.davidpaulpowell.com

LIKE WHAT YOU READ?
SHARE ON SOCIAL MEDIA!

202 - TRANSFORM YOUR MIND, TRANSFORM YOUR WEIGHT

www.ingramcontent.com/pod-product-compliance
Lightning Source LLC
Chambersburg PA
CBHW060848280326
41934CB00007B/965